Disorders of the Cervical Spine

Disorders of the Cervical Spine

Second Edition

edited by

Eurig Jeffreys FRCS

Orthopaedic Surgeon Emeritus, The Robert Jones
and Agnes Hunt Orthopaedic Hospital, Oswestry, UK

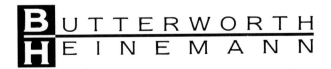
BUTTERWORTH
HEINEMANN

Butterworth-Heinemann Ltd
Linacre House, Jordan Hill, Oxford OX2 8DP

A member of the Reed Elsevier group

OXFORD   LONDON   BOSTON
MUNICH   NEW DELHI   SINGAPORE   SYDNEY
TOKYO   TORONTO   WELLINGTON

First published 1980
Second edition 1993
© Butterworth-Heinemann Ltd 1993

British Library Cataloguing in Publication Data
Disorders of the Cervical Spine. – 2Rev. ed
  I. Jeffreys, Eurig
  616.73

ISBN 0 7506 1361 0

Library of Congress Cataloguing in Publication Data
Disorders of the cervical spine/edited by Eurig Jeffreys. – 2nd ed.
  p.   cm.
  Rev. ed of: Disorders of the cervical spine/Eurig Jeffreys, with
  a contribution by Terrence McSweeney.
  Includes bibliographical references and index.
  ISBN 0 7506 1361 0
  1. Cervical vertebrae – Surgery. 2. Cervical vertebrae – Diseases.
  I. Jeffreys, Eurig. Disorders of the cervical spine.
  [DNLM: 1. Cervical Vertebrae. 2. Spinal Diseases. WE 725 D612
  1993]
  RD533.D573 1993   92–48341
  616.7'3–dc20   CIP

Composition by Scribe Design, Gillingham, Kent
Printed and bound in Great Britain by The Bath Press, Avon

Contents

Contributors

David Jaffray, FRCS
Consultant Orthopaedic Surgeon and Assistant Director of Clinical Studies, The Robert Jones and Agnes Hunt Orthopaedic Hospital, Oswestry, UK

Eurig Jeffreys, FRCS
Consultant Orthopaedic Surgeon Emeritus, The Robert Jones and Agnes Hunt Orthopaedic Hospital, Oswestry, UK

Iain W. McCall, FRCR
Consultant Radiologist, The Robert Jones and Agnes Hunt Orthopaedic Hospital, Oswestry, UK

Robert G. Pringle, FRCS
Consultant Orthopaedic Surgeon, The Midlands Centre for Spinal Injuries, The Robert Jones and Agnes Hunt Orthopaedic Hospital, Oswestry, and The Royal Shrewsbury Hospital, UK

Preface

There have been many advances in diagnostic imaging and surgical techniques since the first edition of this book was published. Iain McCall and David Jaffray have written up to date chapters on these subjects. Robert Pringle has succeeded Terence McSweeney as the Orthopaedic Consultant to the Midlands Centre for Spinal Injuries, and has written on Fractures and Dislocations. He has also added a chapter on Cervical Orthoses.

Preface to the first edition

'Behold, my desire is, that the Almighty would answer me and that mine adversary had written a book.'

Job, XXI, 35.

The cervical spine offers common ground for the orthopaedic surgeon, the neurologist, the neurosurgeon, the rheumatologist, the radiologist and the general physician. I have tried to write a brief survey of the area which I hope will be of some value to all these specialities. Inevitably the book has an orthopaedic accent, and I would like to think that orthopaedic residents in training will find it most useful. I have been selective in my material, and specialists in other fields will be well aware of deficiencies; but they may feel compensated by appreciating some of the orthopaedic problems of managing cervical injury and disease. I have also been selective in my bibliography, confining myself to those references which will lead the interested reader to other sources.

There is no orthopaedic consensus at Oswestry. We are a group of individual surgeons whose orthopaedic philosophies range from the reactionary to the revolutionary. The opinions expressed in this book therefore, are mine. Those opinions however have been moulded by my colleagues, who have criticized my views, rearranged my thoughts, influenced my surgical judgement and taught me.

TEJ
Wrexham
Oswestry

Acknowledgements

The authors are grateful to the Department of Medical Illustration at Oswestry, and to Mr Peter Cox, for the illustrations. The portrait of Richard III is shown by kind permission of the National Portrait Gallery. Mr C.W. Weatherley, FRCS lent X-ray films for the cases illustrated in Chapter 10.

Invaluable help in the preparation of Chapter 5 was given by Mr John Kirkup, FRCS, Archivist to the British Orthopaedic Association, Dr D. Chopin of the Institut Calot, and the Librarians of the Royal College of Surgeons, the Lord Mayor Treloar's Hospital and the Robert Jones and Agnes Hunt Orthopaedic Hospital.

Christine Watkins typed the first edition. She has remained indefatigable in processing, and reprocessing, and reprocessing, this manuscript.

Dr Geoffrey Smaldon, of Butterworth-Heinemann, has encouraged and stimulated us through periods of inevitable, but frustrating delay. We owe him our particular gratitude.

1 Applied anatomy

'Was common clay ta'en from the common earth,
Moulded by God, and tempered with the tears
Of angels to the perfect shape of man.'
                                    'To -' Tennyson 1851.

Introduction

The cervical spine conveys vital structures from and to the head and trunk. It enables the head to be placed in a position to receive from the environment all information other than that provided by touch. We need to know as much as possible about these structures, about movement of the head relative to the neck, and the neck relative to the trunk; disorders of the cervical spine will affect one or other of these things.

Surface anatomy

Many of the important structures of the neck can be seen and felt in the thin patient. Less is apparent in the obese, pyknic individual with a short neck, but certain landmarks can always be found.

The sternomastoid muscle, running from one corner to the other of a quadrilateral area, formed by the anterior midline, the clavicle, the leading edge of the trapezius and the mastoid–mandibular line, divides the side of the neck into anterior and posterior triangles (Figure 1.1).

The posterior triangle contains little which is visible on inspection. Palpation of the base of the triangle (which is really a pyramid) finds the first rib, crossed by the subclavian artery, the lower trunks of the brachial plexus and perhaps a cervical rib or its fibrous prolongation. Higher, the accessory nerve, running

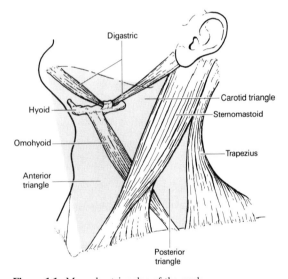

Figure 1.1. Muscular triangles of the neck.

forwards to the sternomastoid, divides the triangle into an upper 'safe', and a lower 'dangerous' area (Grant, 1951).

There is more to be seen, and felt, in the anterior triangle. The external jugular vein, and the platysma, cross the sternomastoid; and both stand out in the thin singer. The 'Adam's apple'* moves with swallowing, and the pulsation of the carotids is often visible. Below the body of the hyoid, the neurovascular bundle

*So called because the forbidden fruit was supposed to have stuck in Adam's throat. There is no canonical authority for this legend. Indeed, Genesis implies that he enjoyed it; and discovered sex.

can be compressed against the carotid tubercle of the sixth vertebra; demonstrating how easily accessible is the spine through this area. In the apex of the triangle, the transverse process of the atlas is palpable immediately behind the internal carotid artery; and the fingertip can roll over the tip of the styloid process and the stylohyoid ligament. In the anterior midline can be usually seen, and always felt, the anterior arch of the hyoid, the notch of the thyroid cartilage, the cricoid and the upper rings of the trachea. With advancing age, the horizontal creases in the skin become more pronounced. Whenever possible, operative incisions should occupy one of these creases, in the interests of healing, if not beauty.

The vertebra prominens, which may be the spinous process of the seventh cervical or the first thoracic vertebra, marks the lower end of the midline sulcus formed by the ligamentum nuchae in its leap to the occiput. The rounded ridge on either side of the sulcus is made by splenius capitis as the origin of trapezius is tendinous. The vertebra prominens is the tip of the 'dowager hump' seen in women with osteoporosis.

The cervical vertebrae

The atlas

The atlas has no body (Figure 1.2). The anterior arch is faceted to receive the tip of the odontoid process, and the medial aspect of each articular mass is indented by the attachment of the transverse band of the cruciate ligament. The spinal canal at this level is spacious. Its sagittal diameter may be divided

into three; the anterior third being occupied by the odontoid peg; the middle third by the cord; and the posterior third by the subarachnoid space. Cisternal puncture by the posterior or lateral route is therefore safe under normal conditions.

The oblique groove across the posterior arch of the atlas accommodates the vertebral artery after it has wound around the outside of the articular mass. The attachment of the posterior atlanto-occipital membrane is arched over the artery at this point, and this arch is sometimes outlined, completely or incompletely, by bone, to form the arcuate foramen. This bony arch is insignificant; but it has been said that its presence renders the atheromatous vertebral artery more vulnerable to compression during rotation of the head (Klausberger and Samec, 1975).

The side-to-side width of the atlas is greater than that of any other cervical vertebra, to increase the leverage of the muscles inserted into the transverse process. This transverse process is the only one in the cervical spine which is not grooved to allow egress of a nerve root. The articular masses are broader and deeper than any other because they shoulder the weight of the skull and because the odontoid process bears no weight.

The axis

The axis has stolen the body of the atlas (Figure 1.3) to form the odontoid peg which projects up from its centrum to lie behind the arch of the atlas. The tip of the odontoid is faceted in front to mate with its atlantic fellow, and behind to accommodate the synovial bursa

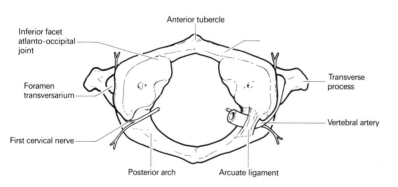

Figure 1.2. Atlas. Superior aspect.

Inferior facet atlanto-occipital joint

Anterior tubercle

Foramen transversarium

Transverse process

First cervical nerve

Vertebral artery

Posterior arch

Arcuate ligament

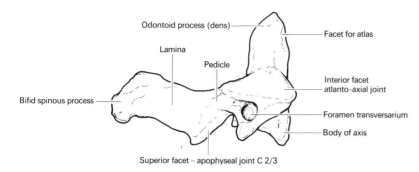

Figure 1.3. Axis. Lateral aspect.

which separates it from the transverse band of the cruciate ligament. On either side of the base of the odontoid, the centrum presents the inferior facets of the atlanto-axial joints. Below, the atlas begins to take on the characteristics of a typical cervical vertebra. Its laminae meet to project a bifid and massive spinous process whose depth and aquiline profile are very variable. The pedicles are thick and their upper margins continuous with that of the body. The inferior articular facet lies below and behind the superior, and subtends an angle of almost 90° with the transverse process. This articulotransverse angle is recessed at its apex to accommodate the tip of the pyramidal process of the third vertebra (Veleanu, 1975).

Vertebrae three to six are so similar that it is not easy, or necessary, to identify an individual bone (Figure 1.4). In the articulated column they increase in size from above downwards. The margins of the bodies are sharply defined, particularly around the superior rim where the posterolateral edge projects upwards to articulate with the body above. Gray does not give this projecting edge a discrete name (Gray's Anatomy, 1969), but Frazer calls it the neurocentral lip (Frazer, 1958), and European anatomists refer to it variously as the unciform or uncinate process, or the semilunate process. It is a structure of sufficient identity to deserve a name, and it is a significant structure in the pathology of cervical spondylosis. In this book it will be referred to as the neurocentral lip. The antero-inferior margin of the body projects downwards. This normal epinasty increases with the development of spondylotic osteophytes, a point to be remembered during discography and anterior interbody fusion.

The spinal canal is large to accommodate the cervical enlargement of the cord. The laminae are slender, and in youth each slightly overlaps the one below. This overlap increases markedly with age.

The pedicles, apophyseal joints, transverse processes and neurocentral lips are peculiar and specific to the cervical spine (Figure 1.5). Together they constitute the boundaries of the

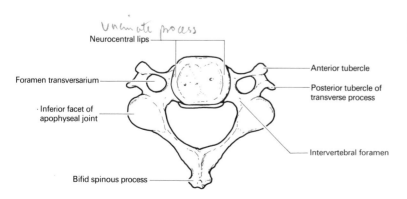

Figure 1.4. Typical cervical vertebra. Superior aspect.

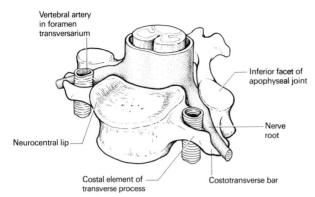

Vertebral artery
in foramen
transversarium

Inferior facet of
apophyseal joint

Nerve
root

Neurocentral lip

Costal element of
transverse process

Costotransverse bar

Figure 1.5. Relations in the intervertebral funnel.

intervertebral foramen and enclose the foramen transversarium. This foramen, which affords passage to the vertebral artery, separates the costotransverse bar from the pedicle. The groove which forms the floor and walls of the intervertebral foramen, becomes progressively more shallow as the vertebrae descend. Medial to the vertebral artery the groove is floored by the pedicle. Here lie the anterior root of the spinal nerve and the posterior root ganglion; the former usually, though not invariably, above the latter (Abdullah, 1958). Running above the nerve root are the radicular and spinal branches of the vertebral artery, and their accompanying veins. Tapering into the groove are the blending layers of the meninges and the nerve sheaths forming the dural root sleeve.

Passing behind the vertebral artery, the spinal root divides. The posterior primary ramus winds around the lateral aspect of the articular mass, or 'pyramidal process' (Veleanu, 1975) and therefore lies behind scalenus medius, which arises from the posterior tubercle of the transverse process. The anterior primary ramus crosses, and grooves the costotransverse bar, and passes between the two scaleni. Given the configuration of the articulated cervical column, it follows that the so-called intervertebral foramen is a funnel at least one centimetre in length and variable in height and width. Its width is determined by the length of the pedicle, and here the funnel is at its most narrow. The walls of the dry bone diverge laterally, but in life only to accommodate the vertebral artery and its surrounding venous plexus. The functional diameter of the funnel may be smaller here than at the pedicle.

The height of the funnel is determined by the height of the articular mass. The tip of this process engages with the apex of the proximal articulotransverse angle. It is subject to normal variations in shape and size, and is also modified with age and the inevitable osteophytic deformation of degenerative spondylosis. Medially, the intervertebral disc, the vertebral body and the neurocentral lip are equally liable to variations in shape and height.

The costal or anterior element of the transverse process, with the side of the vertebral body, forms the floor of the shallow groove which houses longus capitis and longus cervicis muscles. In the muscular man these muscles may extend almost to the midline of the vertebral body, becoming continuous with the anterior longitudinal ligament. When this happens they can be a nuisance during an anterior approach to the cervical spine. On these muscles and anterior to the costal element lies the sympathetic chain, vulnerable to an enthusiastic retractor.

The seventh cervical vertebra is transitional. Its spine is long and not bifid. It ends in a tubercle which affords attachment to the ligamentum nuchae. The spine may or may not be longer than that of the first thoracic vertebra. If it is, the seventh is the vertebra prominens. The transverse processes are large and often lack a foramen transversarium. When one is present, it is traversed by veins and branches of the ascending cervical artery; never by the vertebral artery*. The costal element may be discrete as a cervical rib; a structure whose existence has provoked acrimonious discussion out of all proportion to its size and significance. It is the 'unciform sac' of orthopaedic surgery (Shaw, *The Doctor's Dilemma*).

*'What, never?
Hardly ever.' (HMS Pinafore.)

The joints of the cervical spine

The intervertebral discs

There is no disc between the first and second vertebrae. The odontoid process is separated from the body of the axis by a layer of cartilage which ossifies before puberty. This cartilaginous layer is not an epiphyseal plate but a notochordal remnant. A fracture through the base of the odontoid in childhood is not an epiphyseal injury (Friedberger, Wilson and Nicholas, 1965; Seimon, 1977).

The intervertebral discs are composed of an outer annulus fibrosis containing a nucleus palposus. The posterolateral margins of the annulus lie between the neurocentral lip and the inferior aspect of the body above. After the second decade of life, clefts appear in the annulus in this area. These clefts persist throughout life. They acquire linings indistinguishable from synovial membrane. Adjacent to the clefts, the neurocentral lip develops osteophytic outgrowths similar to the osteoarthritic osteophytes of the apophyseal joint across the pedicle. An academic controversy has existed for many years as to whether these clefts are true synovial joints. The current orthodox teaching is that they begin as stress fissures of the annular fibres, which appear in the second decade of life, and are later converted into cartilage-lined joint surfaces. They are known as the neurocentral joints (of Lushka); or, in European literature, as uncovertebral joints. They are of considerable importance, in the pathogenesis of cervical radiculopathy and myelopathy; and in the operative treatment of cervical myelopathy and the vertebrobasilar syndrome (Von Lushka, 1858; Rathke, 1934; Cave, Griffiths and Whiteley, 1955; Tondbury, 1955; Payne and Spillane, 1957; Ecklin, 1960).

The discs are biconvex to conform with the concavity of the vertebral bodies, but are deeper anteriorly. The normal lordosis of the cervical spine results from this. The nucleus does not occupy the centre of the disc but lies somewhat posterior, a point to remember when performing cervical discography.

The annulus is reinforced in front and behind by fibres from the anterior and posterior longitudinal ligaments. Elsewhere around the circumference of the vertebral body the annulus blends with the periosteum, but is bound down to bone and can only be separated by incision.

The apophyseal joints

These synovial joints lie oblique in the sagittal plane, and incline medially in the coronal. This alignment lacks the architectural stability of the dorsal and lumbar areas of the spine, but permits more movement. A 'fail-safe' locking mechanism is provided by the abutment of the superior leading edge of the inferior facet into the articulotransverse angle of the joint above (Veleanu, 1975). The joint capsules are richly innervated with pain and proprioceptive receptors, more so than in the corresponding joints lower in the spine, so that awareness of head and neck movement is enhanced (Wyke, 1978). Wyke has described three types of nerve endings; types I and II which he refers to as mechanoreceptors, and type III which are nociceptors. His type III receptors are not found in the cervical spine. He also observed that while the apophyseal joint capsule and the supporting ligament of the neck are so innervated, the intervertebral discs are not.

The atlanto-axial and atlanto-occipital joint facets are aligned to permit the movement of nodding and turning peculiar to this level. The atlanto-odontoid joints lie between the facets on the tip of the process and the anterior arch of the atlas in front, and the transverse ligament behind. Two synovial cavities are present, and the posterior articulation is unique in that the facet on the transverse ligament is covered with articular cartilage.

The ligaments of the cervical spine

The occipitovertebral ligaments
(Figure 1.6)

The transverse ligament of the odontoid is diamond shaped and embraces the process securely. Two bands, one passing up to the occiput, the other down to the body of the axis, complete the cruciform ligament of the atlas, but the vertical arms of the cross play little part in containing the odontoid. In front of the upper arm lies the apical ligament of the

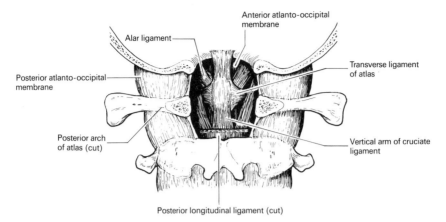

Figure 1.6. Ligaments of the odontoid.

odontoid, a vestigial remnant; and the alar ligaments, running either side from the tip of the odontoid to the margins of the foramen magnum. They are robust cords which check atlanto-axial rotation.

The anterior atlanto-occipital membrane (Figure 1.7) extends upwards from the anterior longitudinal ligament to connect the anterior arch of the atlas with the anterior margin of the foramen magnum.

The membrane tectoria is a fan-shaped continuation of the posterior longitudinal ligament to the basi-occiput. Its superficial lamellae blend with the dura.

The posterior atlanto-occipital membrane arches over the vertebral artery. It is not as strong as the flavum, and during cisternal puncture the advancing needle does not encounter the characteristic 'brown paper' resistance felt during lumbar puncture.

The longitudinal ligaments

The anterior longitudinal ligament hugs the front of the vertebral bodies and loosely blends with each annulus as it crosses the disc spaces. The posterior ligament is firmly bound to each disc, but stands proud of the posterior concavity of the vertebral body. The space is occupied by the retrocorporeal veins. By standing away from the back of the vertebral body, the posterior ligament ensures that the spinal canal is a smooth-walled tube. This also means that any pathological thickening, such as is seen in ossification of the ligament, will compromise the capacity of the canal even in the absence of any spondylotic protrusion of the disc.

The posterior ligaments

The ligamentum flavum is strong and elastic. It extends around the neural arch from the capsule of the apophyseal joint to where the laminae fuse. It is attached to the lower part of the anterior surface of the lamina above and to the upper edge and posterior surface of the lamina below. The ligamentum nuchae runs from the vertebra prominens to the occiput. It is inelastic and can be regarded as the posterior edge of the interspinous ligament, which is an intermuscular septum providing origin for

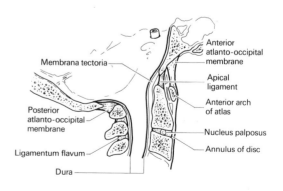

Figure 1.7. Sagittal section of the atlantoaxial joint.

the trapazius and splenius muscles. The inter-transverse ligaments are virtually non-existent in the neck.

Movements of the cervical spine

The erect posture, binocular vision and cervical mobility of humans enable them to recognize the enemy beind their shoulders. The ability to gaze up at the stars or peer down a microscope depends on neck movement. Electronic vision may render neck movement evolutionarily unnecessary; and we may be more concerned to restrict neck movement in the age of the automobile than to encourage it; but head and neck movements remain as social signals indicative of mood or emotion.

Movements of the head on the neck, and movements of the head and neck on the trunk can be described separately, and there is some anatomical jusitification for so doing.

Movements of the atlanto-occipital joints

At these joints we nod our heads. The corresponding curved articular surfaces allow a limited range of flexion and extension. The long axes of the joints are set slightly obliquely; both joints act as one and no movement around a vertical axis can occur. Slight curvature in the coronal plane allows a small degree of lateral tilt.

Extension is arrested when the posterior arch of the atlas is trapped between the occiput and the axis, as is lateral tilt. Flexion stops when the posterior ligaments are taut and when the tip of the odontoid (to which the atlas is firmly linked by the transverse ligament) abuts against the anterior margin of the foramen magnum. During both these movements the movement of atlas on axis is insignificant. After atlanto-axial fusion the range of flexion–extension is undiminished.

Atlanto-occipital flexion is powered by the rectus capitis anterior muscle, supplemented by the longus capitus. Extension is produced by the rectus capitis posterior (major and minor); lateral flexion by the rectus capitis lateralis. The semispinalis and splenius capitis, the trapezius and the sternomastoids assist.

Movements of the atlanto-axial joints

The atlas and the occiput rotate as one around the odontoid. All three atlanto-axial joints take part in the movement. The odontoid is firmly united to the occiput by the alar ligaments which, together with the joint capsules of the atlanto-axial apophyseal joints limit rotation to some 45°.

The muscles producing this rotation are the obliquus capitis and the rectus capitis posterior major, assisted by the splenius capitis of the same side and the sternomastoid of the opposite side.

It can be seen that the strong connections are between atlas and axis, and axis and occiput. Some anatomists even regard the atlas as a mere sesamoid between the skull and the axis, and certainly the occipito-axial-atlantic complex is a functional entity (Werne, 1957). Werne regards the whole complex as a ball and socket joint.

Intervertebral movement between C2 and C7

While the range of movement between any two cervical vertebrae is not great, the summation of these movements provides for the wide range of movement possible in the intact normal neck. The thick intervertebral discs, in the healthy young adult, are compressible and deform to accommodate the range made possible by the flat, upward obliquity of the apophyseal joints.

It is convenient to analyse movement of the whole cervical spine in terms of the spinal motion segment (Ehni, 1984; Giland and Nissan, 1986), that is to say, the articulating unit comprised by two vertebrae, their three joints and their supporting ligaments (Figure 1.8).

Flexion and extension are free around an axis in the postero-inferior area of the vertebral body. Arrest of both is inflicted by bone. Extension is stopped by the contact of superior or inferior facets; flexion by the apposition of the projecting lower edge of the body above on the sloping upper surface of the body below. Lateral flexion is always accompanied by rotation, thanks to the slight medial inclination of the superior facets. This movement is

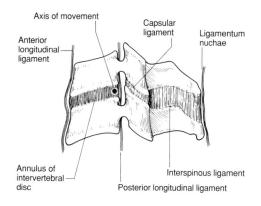

Figure 1.8 The motion segment.

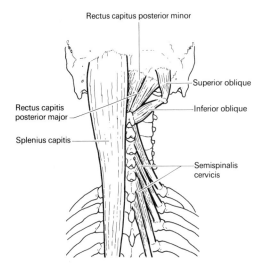

Figure 1.9. Posterior cervical muscles.

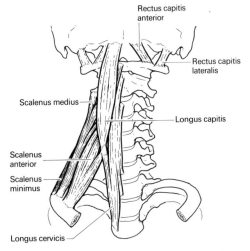

Figure 1.10. Anterior muscles of the cervical spine.

stopped by the lateral locking mechanism of the apex of the inferior facet engaging the transverse-articular angle above.

If bony architecture was the only limiting force in neck movement, control would be vested in the acting muscles alone. Restriction is supplemented by the elastic restraining properties of the two longitudinal ligaments, the ligamentum flavum and the intervertebral discs.

Neck movement diminishes with age. In childhood the free range of flexion and extension can be such as to allow considerable displacement of one vertebral body upon another (Cattel and Filtzer, 1965, and see Chapter 2).

Forward flexion should normally allow the chin to touch the chest. Extension of the neck, in children and the young adult, can sometimes allow the back of the skull to touch the back but this is exceptional. Lateral rotation should encompass a 180° arc, and in lateral flexion the ear should touch the shoulder. These movements can be measured accurately by radiographs, when any segmental restriction can also be detected. The detection of restricted movement on clinical examination in one or more than one direction, is a physical sign of value.

There is a commonplace neck movement which has no precise anatomical term. It is the movement of 'craning the neck'*. It is the movement we use, when standing in a crowd, we try to catch a glimpse of a passing celebrity. The· movement involves simultaneous extension of the atlanto-occipital joints, and flexion of the cervical column on the trunk. The muscles responsible are the two sternomastoids acting together, assisted by the rectus capitis posterior major and minor.

These prime movers can act thanks to the bracing effect of the interspinalis, multifidus and intertransverse muscles which telescope

---

*The etymology of 'craning' leads down strange philological paths. It is a British word meaning to stretch one's neck like a crane. The Old English word is 'cran'. There are no cranes in Britain: but they do exist in Jutland and the Friesian coast, whence our Anglo-Saxon invaders came. Native to Britain however, is the heron; whose foward thrust of beak to impale the foolish eel is the exact neck movement under discussion. The Welsh (or British) name for 'heron' is 'garan'. The crane proper is a rare passage migrant from Scandinavia to Spain. 'Crane' has no connection with 'cranium', which comes from the Greek 'kranion'. The Middle English word for the cranium was 'scolle', hence 'skull'.

the flexed lower cervical spine into a rigid tube.

Other muscles acting on the neck, with the exception of those acting on the occipitovertebral complex, span many segments. Some are confined to the neck, some extend from the neck to the trunk, and some are attached to the skull and trunk. They are illustrated in Figures 1.9 and 1.10.

Stability and instability

Stability of the cervical spine can be defined as the maintenance of vertebral alignment throughout the normal range of movement. Instability is the loss of this ability, allowing vertebral displacement. Displacement of one vertebra relative to another places the cervical cord at risk and jeopardizes the spinal cord. McSweeney has suggested that we use 'safe' and 'unsafe' instead of 'stable' and 'unstable'.

The range of movement of the cervical spine is greater than any other spinal area but it is convenient to discuss stability in the context of one articulation unit, the spinal motion segment of two vertebrae, their intervertebral disc and ligaments and their apophyseal joints. It is also necessary to discuss stability above C2, the upper cervical spine, and below C2, the lower cervical spine, separately.

The factors contributing to stability at all levels are: bony, ligamentous and muscular.

1 Stability at the occipito-atlanto-axial joints

Weight is transmitted from the skull, across the atlanto-occipital and atlanto-axial joints. These surfaces are but slightly curved and offer no stability against horizontal forces. Horizontal stability derives from the integrity of the odontoid process and the check ligaments which retains it in relation to the atlas.

The intact odontoid is held in close relation to the anterior arch of the atlas by two ligaments, or groups of ligaments (Figure 1.6). The transverse atlantal ligament passes between the lateral masses of the atlas, and behind the odontoid, holding it against the anterior arch of the atlas while allowing it to rotate. It is strong and is the first line of defence against atlanto-axial subluxation. It is reinforced by the alar ligaments which pass from the tip of the odontoid to the margins of the foramen magnum. They are check reins, designed to limit rotation, and are inadequate to prevent atlanto-axial displacement if the transverse ligament has been ruptured (Werne, 1957; Fielding *et al.*, 1974).

2 Stability in the lower cervical spine

The two column support of the occipito-atlanto-axial complex is converted into a three column structure below C2. Weight is transmitted via the vertebral bodies and the apophyseal joints. This has been likened to a three-legged stool, a very stable structure (Louis, 1987), but the comparison is not exact because the apophyseal joints lie at an angle of 45° to the horizontal. This angle is not as great as in the thoracic (60°) or the lumbar (90°) spine but, nevertheless, vertical force while being compressive to the vertebral body, applies shear to the apophyseal joint. Unfortunately the angle is too shallow to afford much horizontal protection and facet dislocation without fracture is seen in the cervical spine in a way that is not seen below T1. If more than half of one apophyseal joint is destroyed by disease or operation, the remaining joint will fracture under physiological loading and dislocation will occur even in the presence of intact ligaments (Raynor, Pugh and Shapiro, 1987).

Loss of vertebral body mass will permit instability in flexion. Destruction by disease is gradual and the resulting subluxation is also gradual, as is the myelopathy this causes. Sudden onset tetraplegia in such patients is usually due to tumour encroachment on the cord or anterior spinal infarct rather than subluxation.

The ligaments of the 'posterior complex'; the ligamentum nuchae, the interspinous ligaments, the ligamentum flavum and the capsules of the apophyseal joints, act as an elastic check rein to flexion. If they are disrupted, facet dislocation can occur without fracture and because ligaments do not heal as readily as bone unites, such lesions can be persistently unstable.

The intact disc affords some protection against horizontal shear. It is argued that excision of the disc, without interbody osteosynthesis, leads to instability and progressive subluxation. In practice the opposed vertebrae ankylose by bone or fibrous tissue and a stable structure results.

The small muscles below C2, interspinalis and multifidus, play an important part in lower cervical stability. They telescope the column into a rigid tube while craniocervical movement occurs. They augment the passive check rein effect of the ligaments and can be regarded as 'active stabilizers' (Sherk, 1987).

The cervical fascia (Figure 1.11)

Knowledge of the cervical fascia saves the surgeon from becoming lost in the neck. Deep to the platysma, the investing layer is attached above to the occiput and mandible, below to the clavicle. It splits to enclose the sternomastoid muscle. The prevertebral fascia covers the anterior aspect of the vertebral column and the paraspinal muscles. Between these two sheets, the areolar tissue surrounding structures such as the thyroid, and the neurovascular bundle, is condensed into visceral fascial investments, which can be parted by gentle blunt dissection with the finger. The fascial

arrangements are easier to depict than to describe in words, and can be properly appreciated only in the operating theatre.

The spinal cord and its meninges

The cord is invested by the dura, arachnoid and pia mater (Figure 1.12). The dura is closely applied to the posterior longitudinal ligament behind the vertebral body, and blends with the membrana tectoria in the foramen magnum. Elsewhere in the spinal canal it is separated from bone by a space containing little extradural fat and an enveloping plexus of vessels, mostly venous. It follows the spinal roots through the intervertebral foramen into the funnel where it blends with the perineurium of the emitting nerve. Here it is also attached, albeit loosely, to the capsule of the apophyseal joint.

Each dorsal and ventral nerve root penetrates the dura by a separate ostium, so that a dural septum separates each sleeve. These blend into a single envelope just beyond the dorsal root ganglion. Occasionally this penetration, or invagination, of the dura occurs below the relevant foramen. When this occurs the nerve roots, enclosed in their dural

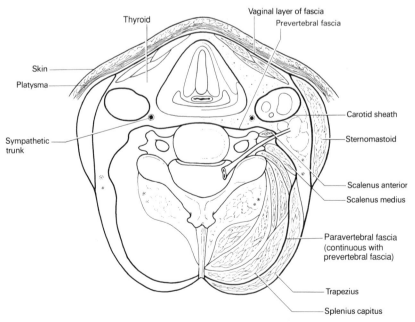

Skin

Platysma

Thyroid

Sympathetic trunk

Vaginal layer of fascia

Prevertebral fascia

Carotid sheath

Sternomastoid

Scalenus anterior

Scalenus medius

Paravertebral fascia (continuous with prevertebral fascia)

Trapezius

Splenius capitus

Figure 1.11. The arrangement of the cervical fascia at the level of C5.

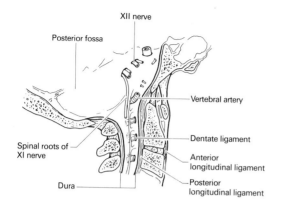

Figure 1.12. The interior of the upper cervical dura.

sleeves, enter the foramen over its lower edge. The angulation of the roots is at the dural ostia. Such angulation is more common in the lower cervical spine and becomes more frequent with advancing age (Frykholm, 1951; Reid, 1958; Abdullah, 1958; Adams and Logue, 1971; Sunderland, 1974).

The arachnoid is applied to the dura and is invaginated with it by the emerging nerve roots. The pia is closely applied to the cord and roots. The dentate ligament is attached to the arachnoid longitudinally between the dorsal and ventral roots and passes laterally to the dura to which it is fixed by a number of triangular (or tooth-like) processes. After cervical laminectomy, the dentate ligament must be divided if the anterior aspect of the cord is to be inspected.

When the neck is flexed, the length of the dura equals that of the spinal canal. The canal shortens when the neck extends, and the dura bulges into concertina-like folds (Breig, 1960).

The cervical enlargement of the cord occupies most of the spinal canal except at the level of the atlas. It is oval in cross section and, in addition to carrying much white matter, has a large proportion of grey matter because it gives origin to the cervical and brachial plexuses, as well as accommodating the spinal nuclei of the Vth and XIth cranial nerves (down to the second or third spinal segments). Knowledge of the various ascending and descending tracts in the white matter is of clinical and radiological diagnostic value.

The cord undergoes elastic deformation during flexion and extension of the neck as the spinal canal alters in length (Breig, 1960). To some extent the cord is tethered by the nerve roots as they enter the intervertebral foramina. The blending of nerve sheath and dura in the foramen forms a similar anchor for the dura (O'Connell, 1955). To the extent that the pia and dura are linked by the dentate ligament, cord and dura deform together, but there is no blending between nerve root and dura in the foramen except when there has been adhesive arachnoiditis. The cord has more leeway laterally. Excessive tension on the opposite nerve root (and excessive compression of the ipsilateral vertebral artery) is prevented by the locking mechanism previously described. This delicate balance between freedom and security can too easily be upset by the altered biomechanics of degeneration or the violence of injury.

The upper three or four cervical nerves contribute to the cervical plexus; the lower five and first thoracic to the brachial plexus.

The first cervical nerve arises above its vertebra, but emerges behind its articular mass. The anterior primary ramus then passes forwards under the vertebral artery. The second cervical nerve also emerges behind the articular mass. All other cervical nerves come out in front of their respective joints. This morphological change has led some anatomists to regard the neurocentral lip of the lower cervical vertebrae as an articular process, and the annular cleft associated with it as a synovial joint 'in series' with the atlanto-occipital and atlanto-axial joints.

The posterior primary rami of the first, second and third cervical nerves are called the suboccipital, great occipital and small occipital nerves (Figure 1.13). They convey sensory fibres to the back of the head as far forwards as the vertex of the skull and the angle of the mandible. A vivid description of the area of skin innervated by C2 is given in *Rest and Pain*, and merits full quotation:

'A short time since, a man, who is now undergoing the punishment of penal servitude, attempted to cut his wife's throat. In drawing the razor across her neck, he divided the auricular branch of the second cervical nerve, and gave me the opportunity of ascertaining the distribution of that nerve. My dresser, as well as myself, pricked with a needle over the whole of the auricular surface, and ascertained minutely the precise position of the loss of sensation consequent upon the division of the cervical nerve; whilst the skin

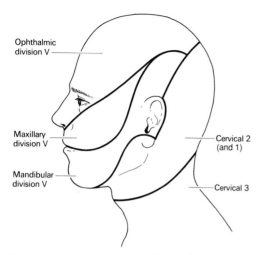

Ophthalmic
division V

Maxillary
division V

Mandibular
division V

Cervical 2
(and 1)

Cervical 3

Figure 1.13. Areas of skin supplied by C1, 2, 3.

which retained its sensation indicated with equal precision the distribution of the fifth cerebral nerve on the external ear.' (Hilton, 1863.)

The brachial plexus is formed from the roots of C5 to T1. A pre-fixed plexus is formed from the lower five cervical roots; a post-fixed plexus from the lower three cervical and the upper two thoracic roots. The lowest trunk of such a formation is said to be vulnerable to compression by a cervical rib or scalenus medius band. Such an anomaly however has little significance in the analysis of cervical root lesions. Innervation of muscle groups by

segments is constant, regardless of which peripheral nerve conveys the axon to its motor endplate (Table 1.1).

The same accuracy cannot be claimed for dermatome charts (Figure 1.14). There is considerable overlap of sensory areas. Further confusion can arise from the appearance of false localizing signs in the early stages of a space-occupying lesion in the upper cervical canal. There may be lack of correlation between motor and sensory levels because of spinothalamic decussation. This should be appreciated, but sometimes a high cervical tumour may cause venous congestion, with resulting hypoxia of lower neurones (Taylor and Byrnes, 1974).

The blood vessels of the cervical spine

The vertebral arteries (Figure 1.15)

The two vertebral arteries contribute between 10 and 15 per cent of the cerebral blood flow (Hardesty *et al.*, 1963). They supply blood to over 90 per cent of the cervical spinal cord, nerve roots and their supporting tissues. Each vertebral artery arises from the subclavian artery. It is uncommon for the two arteries to be the same size. The left is larger than the right in over half the specimens examined; in fewer than one in ten are they the same size. Unilateral, and even bilateral aplasia, have been described (Stopford, 1916; Hutchinson

Table 1.1 Segmental innervation of neck and arm muscles

	Trunk	*Shoulder*	*Arm*	*Forearm*	*Hand*
C1	Deep muscles				
C2	of neck				
C3					
C4	Diaphragm				
C5	Splenius	Rotator cuff	Biceps		
C6	and	and	and brachialis	Extensors and flexors of wrist	
C7	scalenus	deltoid	triceps brachii	Extrinsic extensors and flexors of	
C8				fingers	
T1				Rotators of forearm	Small muscles of hand

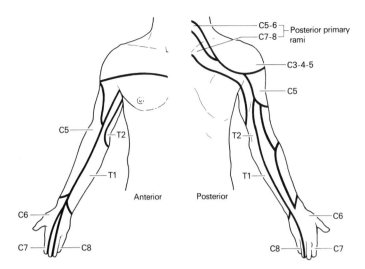

Figure 1.14. Cutaneous dermatomes innervated by the brachial plexus.

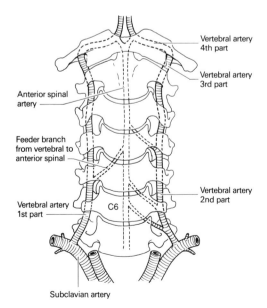

Figure 1.15. Vertebral and anterior spinal arteries.

and Yates, 1956; Tsai *et al.*, 1975; Keller, Meier and Kumpe, 1976). The normal blood flow is towards the skull throughout the cardiac cycle, but reverse flow occurs, fed from the contralateral artery or from the carotid system, when there is stenosis of the subclavian artery proximal to the origin of the vertebral artery. This reversal of flow is known as 'subclavian steal'. In a reported case of bilateral aplasia, the basilar artery was supplied via a dilated branch of the occipital branch of the external carotid. The report does not describe how the anterior spinal system was maintained (Tsai *et al.*, 1975). This left preponderance may explain the greater frequency of clinical syndromes of vertebral artery disease on the left side; but this frequency is far more than can be accounted for on anatomical grounds, and there may well be other reasons (see Chapter 7). The vertebral artery is described in four parts.

The first part runs from the vessel's origin to the apex of the scalene triangle, where it enters the vertebral column through the foramen transversarium of the sixth, rarely the fifth, cervical vertebra. It lies on the transverse process of the seventh cervical vertebra and the lower two roots of the brachial plexus. In front, it is covered by the common carotid artery and vein. The inferior thyroid artery and, on the left, the thoracic duct cross it. The first part may differ in length on each side. It may enter the foramen transversarium of the sixth vertebra on one side, and that of the fifth on the other. Its origin can also vary. The left artery has been seen to arise from the arch of the aorta, on the right from the common carotid and on both sides from the inferior thyroid artery (Abdullah, 1958). No branches arise from the vertebral artery before it enters the bony column.

The second part of the artery traverses the foramina transversarium of the sixth to the first cervical vertebra. Rarely the artery enters the spinal canal below the first vertebra, between the first and second or even the second and third.

Venous plexuses surround the artery in its ascent, and it is accompanied by a branch of the stellate ganglion. The vessel lies immediately behind the anterior root (or costal element) of the transverse process. Medially it is closely related to the vertebral body and the neurocentral lip. Laterally and posteriorly the anterior primary ramus of the particular cervical nerve separates the artery from the posterior bar of the transverse process and the scalenus medius muscle. The pedicle forms the medial margin of the foramen transversarium, and above this the artery comes to lie in front of the ventral root and the dorsal root ganglion of the nerve; the ventral root usually lying slightly below the ganglion. Above again, the capsule of the apophyseal joint is in immediate posterior relation.

As it crosses each nerve the artery gives off anterior, posterior, lateral and medial branches to supply the vertebrae, the intervertebral joints, the adjacent muscles, the nerve roots, the meninges and the spinal cord. Some of these branches anastomose, in the lower part of the neck with branches of the ascending, deep and superficial cervical arteries; and in the upper neck with ascending pharyngeal and occipital branches of the external carotid artery. These anastomoses are rich and abundant (Bowden, 1966; Gooding, 1967; Gooding, Wilson and Hoff, 1975, 1976).

In the normal spine the foramen transversarium lies near the axis of movement in the sagittal plane, so that the second part of the vertebral artery is not compromised during flexion and extension of the neck. In lateral flexion–rotation the locking mechanism of the articulotransverse angle limits movement before the artery on the side to which the movement occurs is compressed, or the contralateral vessel stretched (Veleanu, 1975). These safeguards may fail when the capacity of the intervertebral funnel is diminished by the osteophytic encroachment of cervical spondylosis.

The third part of the artery is described in standard texts as running from the foramen transversarium of the atlas to the point on the posterior arch of the atlas where it passes under the posterior atlanto-occipital membrane

to enter the spinal canal. It would be more logical to regard this section as beginning where the artery leaves the axis. Here it deviates laterally and becomes more liable to be affected by alterations in positions of the head and neck; in health as well as in disease.

Leaving the foramen transversarium of the axis, the artery inclines laterally some 30° to reach the corresponding foramen of the atlas. The anterior ramus of the second cervical nerve emerges lateral to the artery; but the vessel's medial relation is not the vertebral body, but the capsule of the atlanto-axial joint. There is no intervertebral funnel here as the pedicle of the axis lies behind the foramen transversarium. A needle passing over the pedicle, behind the nerve and artery, can easily enter the subarachnoid space. The artery passes through the foramen of the atlas and runs around the lateral aspect of the articular mass to the groove on the posterior arch of the atlas. The first cervical nerve lies between the artery and the bone; the only nerve to pass medial to the vessel. The groove for the artery lies at least one centimetre lateral to the posterior midline tubercle of the atlas, to be remembered when one is passing wires around the posterior arch in atlanto-axial fusion.

The fourth part of the artery, having entered the subarachnoid space, climbs up in front of the roots of the XIIth nerve to the anterior midline of the medulla, and joins its opposite fellow at the base of the pons to become the basilar artery.

The branches of the fourth part of the vertebral artery are the spinal, the medullary and the posterior inferior cerebellar. Such topographical grouping of the artery's branches is artificial. The branches of all parts of the artery are better described as belonging to two groups; those which supply structures in the posterior fossa; and those which supply the cervical cord and its surrounding structures. This second group cannot be considered in isolation from branches of the anastomosing cervical arteries, and will be described together as the extraspinal blood supply of the cord. The intrinsic supply to the cord will be described separately.

Structures supplied inside the cranium

The medullary branches of the vertebral artery supply a small area of the anterior part of the medulla oblongata; the anterior spinal arteries also give branches to the medulla before they unite to form the single anterior midline vessel of the cord. The brainstem area so supplied contains the nucleus of the XIIth nerve.

The posterior inferior cerebellar artery supplies a wedge-shaped portion of the medulla, lying dorsal to the olivary nucleus, with its base lateral; and part of the interior cerebellar peduncle. The structures supplied include the nucleus ambiguus, the nucleus solitarius, the vestibular and cochlear nuclei, the spinocerebellar and lateral spinothalamic tracts, and the upper part of the spinal nucleus of the Vth nerve. Isolated occlusion of the posterior inferior cerebellar artery will produce a characteristic 'lateral medullary syndrome'; but lesions of the vertebral artery itself are more common, when the XIIth nerve nucleus is also affected (see Chapter 6).

Structures supplied in the cervical spine (the extraspinal blood supply of the cord)

Each vertebral artery gives off an anterior, and a posterior, spinal branch. The posterior spinal branch frequently arises from the posterior inferior cerebellar. The anterior branches meet in the midline to form the anterior spinal artery, which runs down in front of the anterior midline sulcus of the whole length of the spinal cord. It receives contributions segmentally at intervals from the vertebral, intercostal and lumbar arteries.

The posterior spinal branches divide on either side to form two posterior spinal arteries, which pass down on the posterolateral aspect of the cord in front of, and behind the dorsal nerve roots. The cervical arteries contribute to these posterior vessels, and the anterior and posterior channels anastomose on the surface of the cord. There is no connection between the two systems inside the cord.

Variations from this standard description are so common that it is hardly possible to say what is normal. There may be but one anterior spinal branch, from right or left. The two branches may differ in size. This is not surprising when one considers the variations of the parent vessels. In nineteen specimens examined by Abdullah, she found nine in which the two sources were equal (Brain and Wilkinson, 1967). Sometimes two paired

arteries–developmental remnants–are found. Similar anomalies are as frequent in the posterior longitudinal system (Dommisse, 1974).

These longitudinal channels are reinforced by segmental branches from the vertebral and cervical arteries (in the cervical spine). These segmental feeder vessels are also subject to wide variation in number and level. There may be none; there may be paired branches at each segment. In one series 62 per cent received anterior medullary feeders at the C4/5 and C5/6 levels, but 12 per cent received none in the cervical spine (Rovira, Torrent and Ruscalleda, 1975).

While contributions from, and anastomoses with, the cervical and external carotid systems do occur, it is the vertebral artery which is the most important source of blood to the anterior spinal artery, the nerve roots, the meninges and the vertebrae. At each intervertebral funnel branches arise. Liable as it is to be affected by disease, this point has been aptly described as 'critical' (Gooding, 1967). From the vertebral arteries anterior and posterior radicular branches run in front of the nerve roots. These branches are constant, and it is important to distinguish them from the variable branches which pass in to reinforce the anterior spinal artery. There has been some confusion, as much over terminology as over description. It has been said that the anterior spinal artery is fed by radicular branches at all levels of the cord (Brain and Wilkinson, 1967). Gray states that some radicular branches, varying in number from four to nine, pass on to join the anterior spinal artery (Gray's Anatomy, 1969). But Dommisse (1974) is clear in differentiation between radicular branches and anterior medullary feeders. There is no doubt but that radicular branches are constant, and contribute to the pial anastomosis on the surface of the cord; but it seems equally certain that contributions to the anterior spinal artery, and therefore to the intrinsic supply of most of the cord, are irregular and infrequent.

Other branches of the vertebral artery arising at the distribution point in the intervertebral funnel, supply the vertebral bodies, the neural arches and the adjacent muscles. These branches anastomose freely with neighbouring segments, and with extravertebral sources.

The intrinsic blood supply of the spinal cord
(Figure 1.16)

The greater part of the interior of the spinal cord is supplied by branches of the anterior artery which penetrate the anterior median sulcus. There is some vertical anastomosis between these branches, but not with the penetrating vessels of the pial anastomosis, which nourish the peripheral parts of the white matter; or with the branches from the posterior spinal arteries within the cord.

The venous drainage of the cervical spine

The intrinsic venous drainage of the cord does not mirror the arterial system, except in the white matter where the drainage is circumferentially into the anterior spinal vein. The grey matter has a separate system, draining upwards from T1 to C2. The two halves of the grey matter have discrete systems (Turnbull, Breig and Hassler, 1966; Gillialan, 1970; Taylor and Byrnes, 1974).

The veins of the vertebral column form a continuous series of plexuses lying in the extradural space. The importance of this plexus in the spread of malignant disease has long been known (Batson, 1940). This plexus is in direct communication at every level with the caval or azygos systems. Most of the cervical spinal drainage is to the confluence of sinuses at the basi-occiput, rather than to segmental veins (Dommisse, 1974).

Changes in the cervical spine due to normal ageing

The body begins to degenerate as soon as it stops growing. Nowhere is this process more apparent than in the spine; as though Nature were exacting retribution for our presumption in standing on our feet. The intervertebral disc, in particular, seems to be phylogenetically unsuited to its role as a weight carrier. Its function in this respect was first recognized by Monro (the founder of that extraordinary dynasty which dominated the study of anatomy in Edinburgh in the eighteenth and nineteenth centuries) in 1771. Arbuthnot Lane described cervical spondylosis in 1886, but it

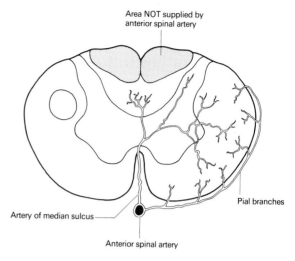

Figure 1.16. Intrinsic blood supply of the spinal cord.

was not until the 1950s that detailed attention was paid to the natural history of ageing in the cervical spine (Hirsch, Schajowicz and Galante, 1967).

The outer layers of the annulus fibrosus receive a scanty blood supply from surrounding vessels, but the inner layers of the annulus and the nucleus palposus are avascular, and incapable of healing after injury. The posterior rim of the annulus is thinner than the anterior (Bowden, 1966), and it is here, and posterolaterally that the disc begins to fissure, probably in the second decade of life. These fissures permit the invasion of vascular granulation tissue. The adjacent bone produces reactive osteophytes. The nucleus becomes desiccated with advancing age and the mechanics of the affected spinal segment are altered, with resulting loss of movement and compensatory increased movement in neighbouring segments, in turn accelerating similar changes there. The osteophytes may encroach on the intervertebral foramen, the exuberant granulation tissue fibroses and may constrict the adjacent nerve roots. The stage is set for the development of the various clinical syndromes associated with cervical spondylosis.

The border between 'normal' degeneration and degenerative 'disease' is difficult to define. A more detailed analysis of the part played by the structural changes of the ageing spine in the pathogenesis of cervical radiculopathy or myelopathy, is deferred until Chapter 7.

References

Abdullah, S. (1958) Quoted by Bowden R.E.M. (1966) in The applied anatomy of the cervical spine and brachial plexus. *Proceedings of the Royal Society of Medicine*, **59**, 1141–1146.

Adams, C.B. and Logue, V. (1971) Studies in cervical spondylotic myelopathy. *Brain*, **94**, 587–594.

Batson, O.V. (1940) Function of vertebral veins and their role in spread of metastases. *Annals of Surgery*, **112**, 138–149.

Bowden, R.E.M. (1966) The applied anatomy of the cervical spine and brachial plexus. *Proceedings of the Royal Society of Medicine*, **59**, 1141–1146.

Brain, Lord and Wilkinson, M. (1967) *Cervical spondylosis and other disorders of the cervical spine* Wm Heinemann Ltd., London.

Breig, A. (1960) *Biomechanics of the central nervous system*. Almgvist and Wiksell. Stockholm, pp 94, 95, 115, 116.

Cattel, H.S. and Filtzer, D.L. (1965) Pseudosubluxation and other normal variations of the cervical spine in children. *Journal of Bone and Joint Surgery*, **47A**, 1295–1309.

Cave, A.J.A., Griffiths, J.D. and Whiteley, M.M. (1955) Osteoarthritis deformans of Lushka joints. *Lancet*, **i**, 176–179.

Dommisse, G.F. (1974) In *Scoliosis and muscle*. (Zorab P., ed). Wm Heinemann Ltd., London, pp 24–36.

Ecklin, V. (1960) *Die Altersveranderungen der Halswirbelsaule*. Springer Verlag, Berlin.

Ehni, G. (1984) Cervical arthroses. *Year Book*. Medical Publishers Inc., Chicago.

Fielding, J.W., Cochran, G.V.B., Lansing, J.F. and Hohl, M. (1974) Tears of the transverse ligament of the axis. *Journal of Bone and Joint Surgery*, **56A**, 1683–1691.

Frazer, J.E. (1958) In *Anatomy of the Human Skeleton*. 5th edn. (A.A. Breathnack, ed) J & A. Churchill Ltd. London, pp 22–23.

Friedberger, R.H., Wilson, P.D. and Nicholas, J.A. (1965) Acquired absence of the odontoid process. *Journal of Bone and Joint Surgery*, **47A**, 1231–1236.

Frykholm R. (1951) Lower cervical vertebrae and intervertebral discs. *Acdta Chirurgica Scandinavica*, **101**, 345–359.

Giland, I. and Nissan, M. (1986) Geometric relations of human cervical spine. *Spine*, **11**, 155–157.

Gillialan, L.A. (1970) Veins of the spinal cord. *Neurology Minneapolis*, **20**, 860–868.

Gooding, M.R. (1967) In *Cervical Spondylosis*. (Brain, Lord and Wilkinson, M., eds) Wm Heinemann Ltd. London, pp. 86–89.

Gooding, M.R., Wilson, C.B. and Hoff, J.T. (1975) Experimental cervical myelopathy. *Journal of Neurosurgery*, **43**, 9–17.

Gooding, M.R., Wilson, C.B. and Hoff, J.T. (1976) Experimental cervical myelopathy: anteroradiographic studies of spinal cord blood flow pattern. *Surgical Neurology*, **5**, 233–239.

Grant, J.B. (1951) *A Method of Anatomy*, 4th edn. Bailliere, Tindall and Cox, London, p. 695.

Gray's Anatomy. (1969) 34th edition. (D.V. Davies and R.E. Coupland, eds). Longman, London, p. 27.

Hardesty, W.H., Whitacre, W.R., Toole, J.F., Randall, P. and Royster, H.R. (1963) Vertebral artery blood flow. *Surgery, Gynecology and Obstetrics*, **110**, 662–664.

Hilton J. (1863) In *Rest and Pain*. 6th edn. (E.W. Walls and E.E. Philipp, eds). G. Bell and Sons, London, p. 73–75.

Hirsch, C., Schajowicz, F. and Galante, J. (1967) Structural changes in the cervical spine. *Acta Orthopaedica Scandinavica*, Suppl. 109.

Hutchinson, F.C. and Yates, P.O. (1956) The cervical portion of the vertebral artery. *Brain*, **79**, 319–331.

Keller, H.M., Meier, W.E. and Kumpe, D.A. (1976) Non invasive angiography in vertebral artery disease. *Stroke*, **7**, 564–569.

Klausberger, E.M. and Samec, P. (1975) Foramen Retroarticulare Atlantis und das Vertebralisangiogramm. *Muncheuer Medizinische Wochenschrift*, **117**, 483–486.

Lane, W.A. (1886) Changes produced by pressure in the bony skeleton of the trunk. *Guy's Hospital Reports*, **43**, 321–434.

Louis, R. (1987) Stability of the cervical spine. In *Cervical Spine I*. (P. Kehr and A. Weidner, eds). Springer-Verlag, Vienna.

McSweeney, T. (1980) in *Disorders of the Cervical Spine*, 1st edn. Butterworth-Heinemann, Oxford, p. 54.

Monro, A. (1771) Mechanism of the cartilages between the vertebrae. *Medical Essays and Observations*, 5th edn. Printed by Cadeol, London and Balfour, Edinburgh, pp. 184–187.

O'Connell, J.E.A. (1955) Involvement of the spinal cord by intervertebral disc protrusions. *British Journal of Surgery*, **43**, 225–247.

Payne, E. and Spillane, J.D. (1957) The cervical spine. *Brain*, **80**, 571–596.

Rathke, L. (1934) Zur Normalen and Pathologischen Anatomia der Halswirbalsaule. *Deutsche Zeitschrift für Chirurgie*, **242**, 122–137.

Raynor, R.B., Pugh, J. and Shapiro, I. (1987) Cervical facetectomy and its effect on stability. *Cervical spine. 1*: (Kehr, P. and Weidner, A., eds). Springer-Verlag, Vienna, pp. 51–54.

Reid, J.D. (1958) Ascending nerve roots and tightness of dura mater. *New Zealand Medical Journal*, **57**, 17–26.

Rovira, M., Torrent, O. and Ruscalleda, J. (1975) Spinal cord circulation in cervical myelopathy. *Neurology*, **9**, 209–214.

Shaw, G.B.S. (1906) *The Doctor's Dilemma*.

Sherk, H.H. (1987) Stability of the lower cervical spine. In *Cervical Spine I*. (P. Kehr and A. Weidner, eds). Springer-Verlag, Vienna.

Seimon, L.P. (1977) Fracture of the odontoid process in young children. *Journal of Bone and Joint Surgery*, **59A**, 943–947.

Stopford, J.S.P. (1916) The anatomy of the vertebral arteries. *Journal of Anatomy of London*, **50**, 131.

Sunderland, S. (1974) Mechanisms of cervical nerve root avulsion. *Journal of Neurosurgery*, **41**, 705–714.

Taylor, A.R. and Byrnes, D.P. (1974) Foramen magnum and high cord compression. *Brain*, **97**, 473–480.

Tondbury, G. (1955) Zur Anatomie und Entwicklungsgeschichte der Wirbelsaule mit Besonderer Berucksichtigung der Altersveranderungen der Bandscheiben. *Schweitzerische Medizinische Wochenschrift*, **85**, 35, 825.

Tsai, F.Y., Mahon, J., Woodruff, J.V. and Roach, J.F. (1975) Congenital absence of bilateral vertebral arteries. *American Journal of Roentgenology*, **142**, 2, 281–285.

Turnbull, J.M., Brieg, A. and Hassler, O. (1966) Blood supply of cervical spinal cord in man. *Journal of Neurosurgery*, **24**, 951–965.

Veleanu, C. (1975) The cervical locking mechanism. *Morphology and Embryology*, **21** (1), 3–7.

Von Lushka, (1858) *Die Halbegelenke des Menschichen Korpers.* Reimers, Berlin.

Werne, S. (1957) Studies in spontaneous atlas dislocation. *Acta Orthopaedica Scandinavica*, Suppl. 23.

Wyke, B. (1978) Clinical significance of articular receptor systems. *Annals of the Royal College of Surgeons of England*, **60**, 2, 137.

2 Diagnostic imaging of the cervical spine

Iain W. McCall

Imaging has two main contributions to make to the management of patients with injury or disease of the cervical spine. It is essential for the accurate diagnosis and delineation of the extent of the lesion and is important in the continuing assessment of its progress.

There have been a number of recent advances in technology which have provided new methods of imaging the anatomy and pathology of the cervical spine with greater detail and tissue differentiation. Computed tomography (CT) enables the spine to be viewed in an axial mode, which permits the evaluation of the relationship between the neurocentral joints, the dural sac and the nerve roots. The improvement in tissue discrimination gained by CT has now been surpassed by magnetic resonance imaging (MRI), which demonstrates the discs, vertebrae, dural sac and cervical cord as discrete entities allowing their interrelationships to be assessed and pathological processes to be evaluated. While the additional information obtained may make specific diagnosis more frequent, there are many changes which are related to the normal ageing process which do not result in symptoms, and the importance of correlating the clinical and radiological findings cannot be overstressed.

The radiologist must be given all necessary clinical information in order that he or she can advise on the most appropriate imaging method and give an opinion on the result. Consultation between the clinician and the radiologist over problem cases is also extremely valuable so that the information that has been obtained can be assessed in the widest perspective and the applicability to the individual patient of further tests which may be invasive, can be evaluated taking into account the balance of clinical benefit and potential harm. Although these new techniques have resulted in a significant reduction of interventional examinations, such as myelography, their replacement is not, as yet, complete and there remains a requirement to restrict the patient X-ray dose from CT, while both CT and MRI have cost implications. The basic plain X-ray remains the most cost effective and quick method of assessing the bone structures and the related soft tissue changes in the cervical spine and is likely to remain a cornerstone of the initial assessment.

Standard radiography

The standard radiographic views are antero-posterior (AP) (Figure 2.1a) and lateral views (Figure 2.1b) of the cervical spine. The antero-posterior view demonstrates the vertebral bodies, the overlying spinous process and the lateral articular mass. It is particularly useful for showing the neurocentral joints formed by the uncinate process on the lateral aspect of the posterior rim of the vertebral end plates. The lateral view demonstrates the vertebral bodies, facet joints and spinal canal. The spinous processes are also seen well in the lateral view, as is the prevertebral soft tissue.

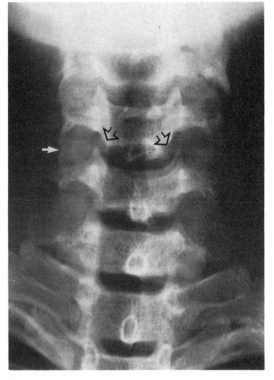

a

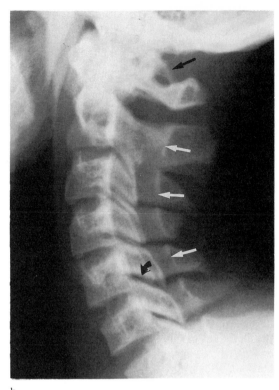

b

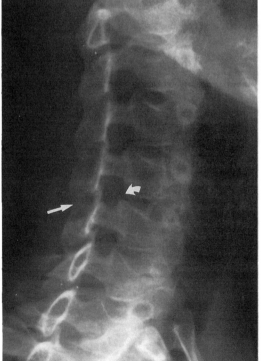

c

Figure 2.1(a). Standard anteroposterior view. The neurocentral joints (⇒), articular mass (white arrow) and transverse process are demonstrated. (b) Lateral view of adolescent. The apophyseal joints, (↗) the spinolaminar line demarcating the posterior margin of the canal (white arrow) and ring apophyses are clearly seen. The arcuate ligament is completely ossified (→). (c) The oblique view at 45° shows the oval intervertebral foramen, the lateral mass and facet joints and the relationship of the neurocentral joints to the foramen (⇒).

The whole cervical spine should be seen adequately on the lateral films, but if the shoulders are heavily built it may be difficult to see the lower cervical vertebrae. Failure to show the whole cervical spine should not be accepted and if traction on the arms does not achieve the objective, a lateral oblique (Figure 2.1c), the so-called swimmer's view, with one arm raised will be required.

The standard AP view may not show the atlanto-axial region and in the circumstances a transoral view will be required (Figure 2.2) although some have suggested that it should not form part of the basic examination (NRPB, 1990).

Oblique views of the lower cervical spine may be performed at 45° and are primarily of value to assess the intervertebral foramen, although the lateral mass and pedicles are clearly demonstrated (Figure 2.1c)

Computed tomography

The physical principles of plain X-rays have been established over the last century and computed tomography remains essentially an X-ray system with sophisticated detectors replacing the X-ray film, allowing digital analysis of the attenuation coefficients of multiple small segments of the tissue being X-rayed. The segment, named pixel, is analysed on a multidirectional basis and the overall image reconstructed pixel by pixel through computer analysis of the numerical values of the attenuation coefficient, which are then related to a grey scale, producing the final image (Figure 2.3). This allows a wide discrimination of tissue densities across the image. The image is then displayed, both on a television system and through a hard copying facility. The sophistication of the equipment has increased over the last 10 years and the speed of imaging and computer analysis has dramatically improved. The digital nature of the imaging information allows data manipulation and thus reconstruction in multiple planes and localized analysis of tissue densities.

Magnetic resonance

This technique exploits the magnetic properties of the hydrogen proton, which under

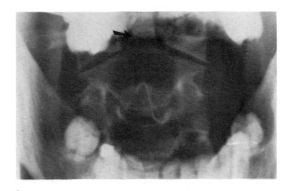

a

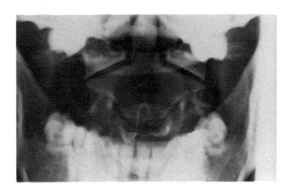

b

Figure 2.2. Transoral view. (a) The apophyseal joints between C1 and C2 are clearly demonstrated and are shown to slope downward in the coronal plane. The odontoid is obscured by the incisor (→). (b) A further view is taken with more tube angulation which now demonstrates the odontoid and reveals a fracture across the base.

carefully defined conditions behaves as a small magnet. Under normal circumstances, the hydrogen protons in the human body have a random orientation so that their small magnetic fields cancel, leaving no net magnetization. If a strong external magnetic field is applied around the body the protons will align themselves along the direction of the field yielding a net magnetization. If further magnetic energy is applied to the protons at right angles to the field via a radiofrequency pulse the angle of net magnetization is altered and the protons absorb energy. Provided no further perturbation occurs, the displaced magnetization will gradually return to the longitudinal axis. During this process the energy given off is a measure of the number of

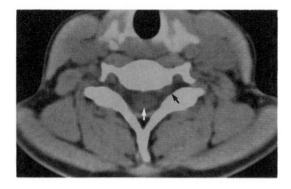

a

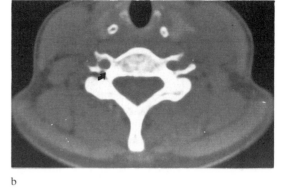

b

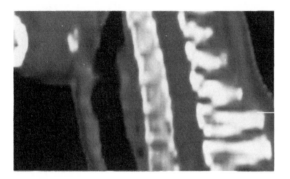

c

Figure 2.3. CT scans of cervical spine. (a) Soft tissue window settings. The cord (⇨) and nerve roots (→) can be visualized. The vertebral artery is also seen in the vertebral canal and the muscles of the neck and main vessels are clearly demonstrated. (b) The bone setting shows the transverse process, (↗) pedicles and lamina. The detail of the spinal canal contents is lost. (c) Reconstruction of the CT images provide a sagittal image of the spine.

nuclei present. The phenomenon of return to equilibrium is termed relaxation and is characterized by two time constants designated T1 and T2. T1 relaxation is termed the longitudinal or spin-lattice relaxation as the nuclei lose the extra energy they gained from the radiofrequency pulse to their local environment. T2 relaxation is transverse or spin-spin relaxation and is a measure of the time required for the spin of the protons, which have been induced to rotate in phase by the radiofrequency pulse, to lose that coherent rotation. T2 reflects a loss of transverse magnetization owing to the interactions of adjacent nuclei.

Both longitudinal and transverse relaxation occur simultaneously but independently and are properties of all normal and pathological tissues and fluids. The relative contribution of each of these properties can be influenced by the choice of pulse sequences.

Image contrast results from a complex relationship between signal intensity, tissue type, specific proton magnetic parameters and the timing characteristics of the pulse sequences. It is also affected by blood flow. The absence of protons in air results in very low signal and if the protons are tightly bound, they have very short relaxation time and no appreciable signal as in tendons or bone. On T1 weighted images, subcutaneous fat and bone marrow have the brightest signal while hyaline cartilage is less bright and muscle even less so (Figure 2.4a). Cystic fluid, urine, ligaments, tendons and bone have little or no signal intensity. On T2 weighted images, however, cystic fluid and urine have the brightest signal followed in decreasing order by subcutaneous fat, bone marrow and muscle (Figure 2.4b). Tumours thus have characteristics which depend on the relative proportion of fat, hydrated tumour cells and fibrosis. Blood flow has special imaging characteristics but in most spin echo sequences major vessels show no signal. In faster gradient echo sequences blood may produce a high intensity signal. The chemical state of the haemoglobin will also affect the imaging appearance in areas of haemorrhage.

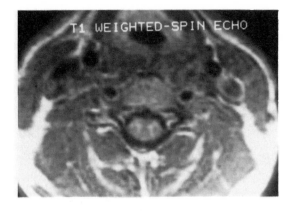

a

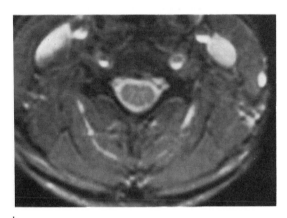

b

Figure 2.4. Axial MRI scan of cervical spine. (a) T1 weighted image showing the cord surrounded by low signal (black) CSF with the nerve roots surrounded by high signal (white) fat. The vertebral arteries are low signal. (b) T2 weighted image. The CSF is now high signal (white). Discrimination of the white and grey matter of the cord is present on both sequences.

Because adjacent normal and pathological tissue can have identical intensities at a given pulse sequence, and thus be obscured, at least two pulse sequences are obtained in most diagnostic examinations.

The choice of pulse sequence is also influenced by the likely localization of a lesion. If it is situated in fat then a T1 weighted examination will produce optimal contrast between the low intensity tissue and the surrounding high intensity fat, whereas if a lesion is located in muscle, which has a relatively short T2 relaxation time, then nearly all pathological process will be of higher intensity.

The presence of metal artefacts can seriously detract from MR images by producing focal loss of signal, often with regional distortion.

The quality of the image is dependent on many parameters including the overall magnet strength, but the design of the receiver coil is very important and specific coils are produced for different anatomical areas.

Radioisotope scanning

Imaging of the cervical spine with a gamma camera following the injection of the isotope technetium-99m labelled with methylene diphosphonate is of value to identify foci of increased bone turnover. The level of isotope uptake is dependent on blood flow, diffusion rates and bone activity. Increased uptake will occur in the presence of increased blood flow and diffusion and this can be assessed by undertaking an early scan at 5 minutes post-injection. The assessment of increased bone activity requires scanning to be undertaken at three hours post-injection when the isotope has been absorbed into the surface of the hydroxyapatite. A number of causes of increased activity in the cervical spine include hypertrophic bone formation of facet osteoarthritis (Figure 2.5), infection or severe degeneration in the discs, Paget's disease and bone producing tumours such as osteoid osteoma and, thus, an increase in activity is not disease specific. The anatomical detail in the cervical spine is less clear when compared with the lumbar spine, due to the reduced size of the vertebrae and the limitations of resolution of the imaging system. The use of emission computed tomography (ECAT) enhances the sensitivity of the system and allows anatomical delineation of the scan in the axial planes. The combination of ECAT isotope and CT scans give a precise diagnosis of lesions such as osteoid osteomas, and other tumours including metastases may be diagnosed in this way (Patton and Woolfenden, 1977).

The presence of infection may be accurately analysed, using other isotopes such as gallium-67 citrate or indium-111. The former is non-specifically absorbed by white cells and by serum proteins, but the latter may be specifically labelled to leucocytes (Merkel *et al.*, 1984). Magnetic resonance has also been

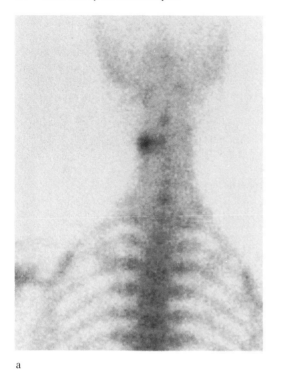

a

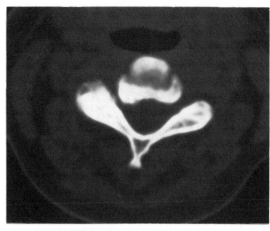

b

Figure 2.5. Tc-99m methylene diphosphonate isotope scan. (a) The normal uptake pattern does not discriminate between individual cervical vertebrae. Localized increase in activity, however, is seen in the lateral mass although the detail is poor. (b) A CT scan of the spine demonstrates hypertrophic bone formation around an osteoarthritic facet.

shown to demonstrate features which indicate the presence of infection and may show changes before an increase in isotope uptake is demonstrated (Szypryt *et al.*, 1988).

Atlanto-axial region

On the lateral view the odontoid lies in close relationship with the anterior arch of the atlas in the adult, with a maximum of 2 mm separation, even on flexion. In the child, greater flexibility is present and 5 mm of separation may be within normal limits. The lateral masses of the atlas are clearly seen on the AP, the lateral views and the flattened angled facet articulation between C1 and C2 is clearly seen on the transoral view (Figure 2.2c). The facet joints at C1/2 and C2/3 are angled downwards and this angulation makes the outline of the facets indistinct on the lateral views, which should not be mistaken for a compression fracture. The anterior arch of the atlas and the incisors may overlap the odontoid on this view and should not be confused with a fracture of the odontoid (see Figure 2.2). Fractures of the odontoid may

be difficult to identify on plain lateral radiographs. Slight movement of the head from side to side during lateral exposure will produce a tomographic effect but linear tomography may prove necessary. CT with 2 mm slices and the reconstruction mode is also effective (Figure 2.6).

CT is the best method to demonstrate the anterior and posterior arches of the atlas and their relationship to the axis in the transaxial plane. This technique should be undertaken for all cases where a fracture of the atlas is suspected (Figure 2.7). The normal anatomical relationship of the skull to the atlas may be assessed on the AP1 by a line across the tips of the mastoid processes. On the lateral view the most commonly used measurement is the McGregor line (McGregor, 1948) which extends along the hard palate to the most caudal margin of the occiput. A similar line to the posterior rim of the foramen magnum was described by Chamberlain (1939) (Figure 2.8). Normally the tip of the odontoid should not project more than 4 mm above this line, although a wide variation according to sex and age has been recorded (Hink, Hopkins and Savara, 1961).

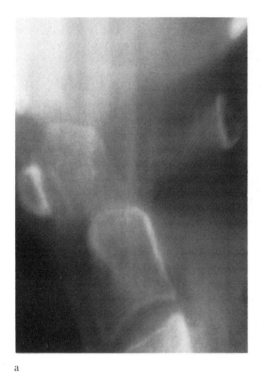

a

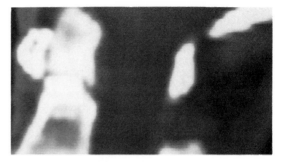

b

Figure 2.6. The fracture of the odontoid is shown clearly on (a) a lateral tomogram and (b) sagitally reconstructed transaxial CT scans.

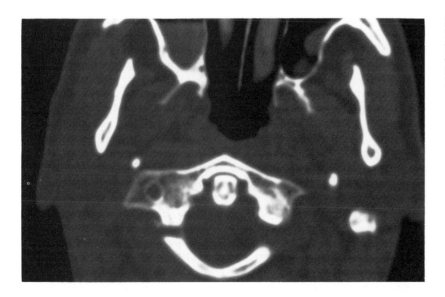

Figure 2.7. CT of atlas. Bilateral wide separation of the lamina of the atlas is demonstrated. Early callus formation is seen on the left.

The relationship of the odontoid to the foramen magnum may be demonstrated more precisely using the reconstruction mode of 2 mm transaxial CT slices through the occipito-atlanto-axial region (see Figure 2.6). The bone structure is well seen on the bone window settings and the relationship to the dural sac can be seen on soft tissue settings. CT is also invaluable in demonstrating the axial relationship between the atlas and axis, in particular the presence of rotational subluxation, which is easy to miss on the AP and

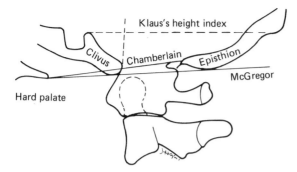

Figure 2.8. Diagnostic lines at the base of the skull.

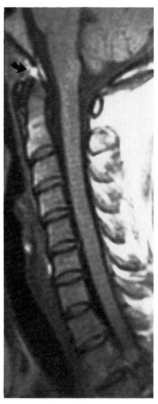

Figure 2.9. T1 weighted lateral MR of the cervical spine. The normal relationship of cervicomedullary junction shows an angle of 170°. A normal small fat pad is seen between the odontoid and the clivus (↖). There is a small disc prolapse at L5/6.

lateral views of the cervical spine. The relationship of the odontoid to the foramen magnum and the cervicomedullary junction is, however, best seen on magnetic resonance (Figure 2.9).

The foramina-odontoid ligament is clearly demonstrated, with an associated fat pad superior to the odontoid, but the transverse ligament cannot be differentiated from the low signal intensity of the posterior cortex of the odontoid. Associated muscle groups can be seen on both CT and MR transaxial scans. The dural sac is demonstrable on the CT scan but the cord cannot be differentiated from the dural sac. The relationship of the uncinate process of the cerebellum to the foramen magnum is easily seen on the centre slices of the magnetic resonance scan, and the pons, medulla and upper cervical cord can all be clearly demonstrated on T1 weighted spin echo (SE) images, surrounded by the dark CSF, which is seen as bright intensity on the T2 weighted SE or gradient echo sequences. The angle of the cervicomedullary cord at the occipito-atlanto-axial junction is normally more than 167° (Figure 2.9).

Congenital anomalies such as Klippel-Feil syndrome and abnormalities which lead to platybasia include cleidocranial dysostosis, osteogenesis, imperfecta, and also conditions which lead to bone softening, such as Paget's disease. In the child the ossification centre of the tip of the odontoid peg may be seen separately and should not be diagnosed as an avulsion fracture. Congenital anomalies in the region of the atlanto-axial articulation involve either hypoplasia of the odontoid peg or failure of ossification of the peg. The former is associated with a number of generalized dysplasias, including trismomy 21 and the mucopolysaccharidoses. Non-fusion of the ossification centre of the peg is demonstrated as an os odontoideum, which may result in a degree of instability of the atlas on the axis (Figure 2.10). The arch of the atlas may also be hypoplasic and this inherent weakness posteriorly may result in increased sclerosis and thickening of the anterior arch. Ossification of the arcuate ligament may be partial or complete and is a normal feature (see Figure 2.1).

Lower cervical spine

The cervical vertebral bodies form the main structure of the anterior spinal column and have a similar anatomy from C3 to C7. The upper end plate is flat, whereas the lower end plate tends to be concave. The bodies become

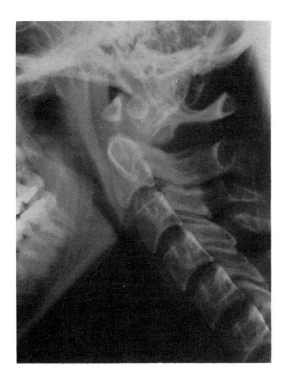

Figure 2.10. Os odontoideum. The round unfused odontoid is seen posteriorly displaced on flexion with the body of C2 anterior to the arch of the atlas.

broader and gradually increase in size from C3 to C7. The intervertebral discs have an outer annulus and central nucleus and the disc is wider anteriorly than posteriorly, producing a lordosis of the cervical spine (see Figure 2.1). The anterior disc space widening is obliterated on flexion. The prominent uncinate processes, on the posterior vertebral rim form the pseudo-articulation, variously known as the neurocentral or uncinate joints or joints of Luschka, which lie close to the intervertebral foramen and the nerve root. Clefts may appear in the posterior annulus laterally, producing a connection between the nucleus and the uncovertebral joints. The pedicles of the cervical vertebrae are short and connect the vertebral body to the articular pillars, mid-way between the superior and inferior articular process. Completing the ring of the canal is a short lamina from either lateral mass, which unites to form the base of the spinous process. This is not well seen on the AP views but is clearly visualized on the transaxial plain by CT (see Figure 2.3).

The tips of the spinous processes are often bifid in the cervical spine and these can be seen on the AP view and CT. The foramina in the transverse processes, which provide for the passage of the vertebral artery can only be demonstrated on CT. The articular mass has a diamond shape on the lateral view and has a rectangular shape on the AP. The intervertebral foramina are demarcated by the pedicle above and below, the uncinate processes anteriorly and the tip of the inferior portions of the lateral masses posteriorly. The close proximity of the uncovertebral joints and the vertebral artery to the nerve roots is clearly demonstrated on the transaxial computed tomogram (see Figure 2.3), which also demonstrates the triangular configuration of spinal canal. The facet joints overlap on the lateral view and, in order to evaluate individual joint spaces, a 10° off lateral view is particularly valuable, especially if minor subluxation or fractures of the facet joints are suspected.

Oblique views at 45° also demonstrate the relationship of the lateral masses and pedicles to each other and should be used in cases of trauma. If significant cervical spinal injury is suspected the oblique views may be obtained with the patient remaining supine but the tube being angled at 45° to the patient (McCall, Park and McSweeney, 1973). Forward displacement of one facet on a neighbour will lead to a break in the line of the lateral masses and alteration of the outline of the foramen from an oval to a

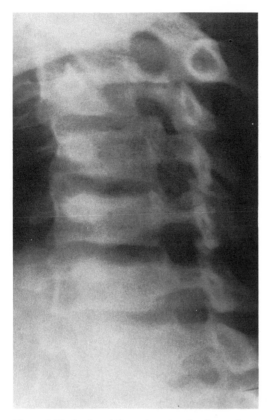

Figure 2.11. Supine oblique view showing forward displacement of C3 on C4, with a kidney-shaped foramen, compared with the normal oval shape of the foramina below.

kidney shape (Figure 2.11). The facet joints may be demonstrated by CT when the relationship is seen as the two joints facing with slightly concave surfaces. If dislocation has occurred, the related surfaces will be convex. Fractures of the facets and adjacent lamina are easily visualized on CT (Figure 2.12), although care must be taken not to misinterpret the partial volume effect of the individual slices at the edges of the lamina, or overlap of lamina as a fracture.

On MR in the sagittal plane the sections pass through the lateral mass and the joint. The lateral mass is seen as a diamond-shaped dark line produced by low signal of cortical bone surrounding the grey area intermediate signal of trabecular bone and marrow. A thin line of lighter tissue may be identified which is the articular cartilage (Figure 2.13). This is not always seen and recent studies with cryomicrotome images have indicated that the resolution is insufficient to show degenerative changes in the majority of cases (Fletcher *et al.*, 1990).

Flexion and extension films are valuable to accentuate relatively occult abnormalities and to assess the effect of obvious lesions. The normal range is usually over 90° and these should be even angulation at each level. Forward displacement of less than 2 mm at a number of levels may be seen in children and some young adults on flexion, producing a step ladder effect. The alignment reverts to normal in extension and these appearances are not found in older subjects. In children, these features may be limited to the C2/3 level, but

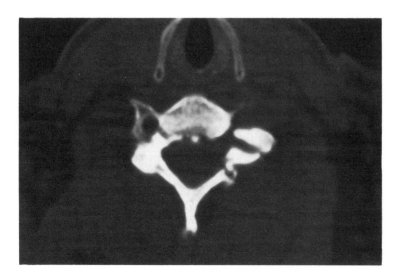

Figure 2.12. Fracture of laminal and articular mass with wide separation of the joint space shown by CT.

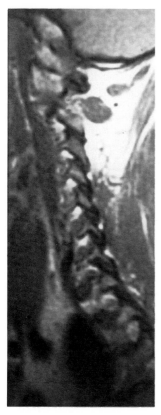

Figure 2.13. T1 weighted MR sagittal image showing the articular processes and facet joints. The intermediate signal of the articular cartilage can be identified. The fat in the intervertebral foramina is seen as high signal.

body and spinolaminar line which represents the junction of the lamina at the base of the spinous process (Tchang, 1974). The sagittal diameter is widest at the C1/2 level with a range of 16–30 mm. In the region of C4 to C7 the range is smaller, between 13 and 22 mm (Burrows, 1963). The sagittal diameter is approximately one half of the coronal diameter, thus encroachment in the sagittal plane will compromise the spinal cord much more quickly than narrowing in the coronal plane. The area of the canal and cord can be measured on CT which will also identify asymmetrical narrowing of the canal. This is difficult to appreciate on the plain AP and lateral radiographs. When the canal is narrowed by osteophyte formation on the posterior rim of the vertebral end plates an accurate measurement can be obtained on the plain lateral films. The degree of narrowing may, however, be underestimated if there is a significant annular bulge or disc prolapse or if there is thickening of the ligamentum flavum which may be especially prominent on extension and cannot be visualized on plain radiographs.

The true AP diameter of the canal, including the soft tissue, can only be assessed accurately on magnetic resonance. The true relationship of the canal diameter to the dural sac is best appreciated on the T2 weighted gradient echo images, where the high signal from the CSF is clearly outlined against the lower signal of the posterior vertebral margin and the ligamentum flavum (Figure 2.15) (Kulkarni *et al.*, 1988).

Widening of the canal may also clearly be appreciated on the lateral view of the cervical spine. The posterior border of the vertebral bodies may be scalloped and the spinolaminal line may be lost or become concave. The appearances may be due to dural ectasia but the presence of an intraspinal tumour must be excluded and this is best undertaken with magnetic resonance. Sagittal and axial T1 weighted images, before and after gadolinium DTPA enhancement, will accurately demonstrate the presence of a tumour and the T2 weighted image will show the effect on the CSF. Myelography is usually unnecessary and may be contraindicated.

The lateral X-ray of the cervical spine will also demonstrate abnormalities of the vertebral bodies. Fusion of vertebrae, due to congenital failure of segmentation may also involve fusion of the posterior elements. The

care must be taken to avoid missing localized trauma (Wakeley, Cassar-Pullicino and McCall, 1991). The facet joints on flexion and extension lateral radiographs have a sliding movement pattern between flexion and extension. In full flexion, the joint surfaces remain parallel but with reduced overlap. In extension, there is anterior widening of the joint space, with narrowing posteriorly (Figure 2.14).

Localized spasm may lead to segmental limitations of movement due to soft tissue trauma. Disc degeneration and narrowing will also limit the range of movement at the affected level but this may cause increased stress above and below these levels and some forward horizontal displacement may occur. The sagittal diameter of the spinal canal can be measured easily on the lateral radiograph between the posterior edge of the vertebral

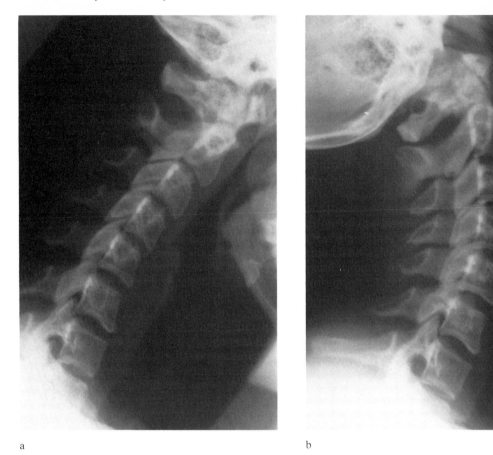

a   b

Figure 2.14. Flexion (a) and extension (b) lateral views demonstrate the sliding motion of the facets. A mild step-ladder effect on flexion is demonstrated, which is resolved on extension.

sagittal diameter of the fused vertebral bodies is reduced, particularly at the disc level. When fusion follows infection, injury or inflammatory diseases such as ankylosing spondylitis or Still's disease, sagittal diameter of the vertebral body is usually normal, especially at disc level. Still's disease affecting young children may, however, prove an exception. Fusion itself does not cause any specific problems but may lead to abnormal stress and early degeneration above and below the lesion and, in the case of ankylosing spondylitis, increases the risk of fracture from minor injury.

Rheumatoid destruction of the discs and posterior joints are well demonstrated by plain radiographs and these changes may result in segmental instability and the forward subluxation of one vertebra on another. Erosion of the odontoid and resultant atlanto-axial or cranio-

caudal subluxation can be clearly demonstrated on plain films but the exact position of the odontoid in the case of upward subluxation is best demonstrated on lateral or computed tomography. Magnetic resonance is, however, the best method of demonstrating the resultant effect on the cervicomedullary junction (Figure 2.16) (Bundschuh *et al.*, 1988), and also demonstrates granulomatous tissue around the odontoid or in the canal, which may be causing increased pressure on the cord (Petterson *et al.*, 1988).

Cervical disc degeneration is a normal ageing process and is present in 80 per cent of Europeans over the age of 60 (Brain, 1962). The plain radiographic features are best visualized on the lateral view and include narrowing of the disc space, with anterior osteophyte lipping due to associated annular bulging. The

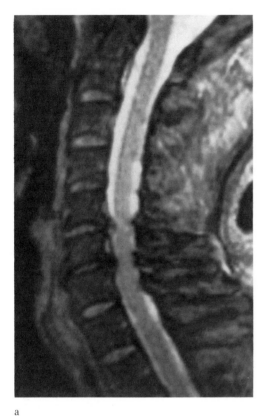

a

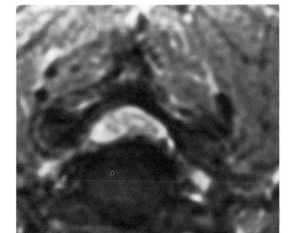

b

Figure 2.15. (a) Lateral T2 weighted MR image, which shows the high signal CSF and intermediate signal of the cord being compressed by a disc prolapse at C5/6 and an osteophyte at C6/7. The ligamentum flavum is also indented, which compounds the degree of compression. (b) The eccentric nature of the compression is shown on the transaxial view.

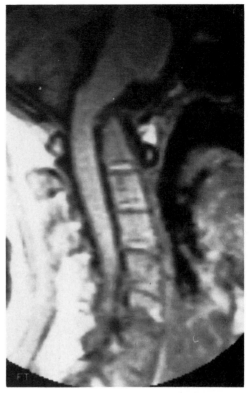

Figure 2.16. T1 weighted MR image shows extensive destruction of the odontoid, with subluxation of C2 into the foramen magnum. The angle of the craniocervical junction is markedly reduced to 125°.

end plates may be sclerotic and occasionally they may appear irregular. Vertebral sclerosis may occur in severe cases. Posterior osteophytes may be present, which are often associated with degeneration at the neurocentral joints, but may also be central at the attachment of the posterior longitudinal ligament. Finally, the picture is completed by the presence of narrowing of the cervical facet joints, with sclerosis of the subchondral bone and often marginal hypertrophic bone formation, best seen on the AP views (Figure 2.17). There is usually a loss of lordosis. Osteoarthritic changes in the facets may also occur at different levels from the disc narrowing, with the former being seen from C2/3 to C4/5 and the latter most commonly at C5/6. This may reflect the lordosis of the cervical spine and the patterns of movement in flexion and extension.

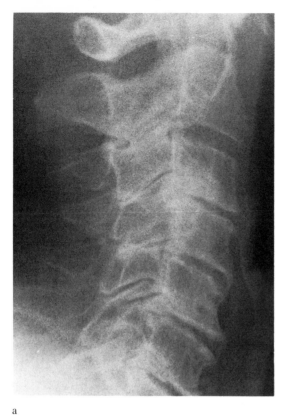
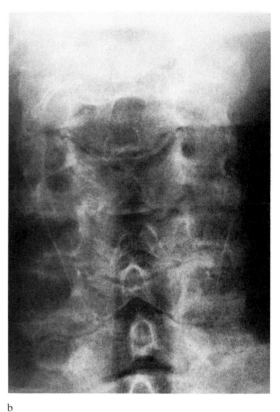

a   b

Figure 2.17. Severe degeneration shown on these lateral (a) and AP (b) views of the cervical spine. Severe disc, facet and neurocentral joint narrowing with adjacent bone sclerosis is seen.

Magnetic resonance scans do not add a great deal of extra information to the basic diagnosis of degeneration. Differentiation of the nucleus from the annulus is not as well demonstrated in the cervical spine compared with the lumbar spine as the disc is generally high signal on T2 and therefore early degeneration is not as easily recognized. Signal reduction may be seen in the marrow of the adjacent vertebral bodies, which will be seen as reduced signal on T1 weighted images due to sclerosis of the vertebral trabeculae. Transaxial images will show the relationship of the cord to the canal. Indentation of the dural sac may be due either to disc prolapse or to osteophyte formation (see Figure 2.15). These are difficult to differentiate on T1, due to the low signal of the CSF and of the osteophyte. The degree of indentation is better evaluated on T2 gradient echo images, where the CSF is a bright signal and the osteophyte is a low signal. In this sequence

the disc prolapse is moderately bright but is outlined by low signal longitudinal ligament and can be differentiated from the dural sac and from osteophytes (see Figure 2.15) (Kulkarni *et al.*, 1988).

The dissociation of clinical and radiological manifestations of cervical spondylosis is well recognized and the rarity of neck pain as a symptom in elderly people contrasts sharply with the degenerate radiological picture. Even the extra detail provided by MR is not symptom-related, with 60 per cent of asymptomatic subjects over 40 years old showing features of degeneration and 28 per cent showing significant lesions such as disc herniation, bulging and foraminal stenosis (Boden *et al.*, 1990). Symptoms, when they occur, are often self-limiting, but in some patients they persist and can be debilitating and further investigation and treatment become warranted.

Cervical myelography

If the clinical picture suggests either a cervical root compression or a cervical myelopathy, further investigation is usually required and the demonstration of the cervical cord and nerve roots by means of intradural water soluble contrast medium has been a major investigative procedure over the last decade. Non-ionic water soluble contrast media are non-neurotoxic and may be introduced into the dural sac either by lumbar or lateral C1/2 punctures. In a recent survey of practice by neuroradiologists 64 per cent regularly injected the contrast by lumbar puncture and 24 per cent by C1/2 puncture (Robertson and Smith, 1990). The former requires between 10 and 15 ml of 300 mg/l injected into the lumbar spine and is carefully manipulated into the cervical spine with the table head down and good cervical extension. The cervical C1/2 injection is undertaken by lateral puncture of the dural sac between the posterior arch of the atlas and the upper surface of the lamina of the axis, where the dural sac is larger and in approximately the posterior third of the canal just posterior to the cord (Cox, Stevens and Kendall, 1981). With the table horizontal and the patient prone 8–10 ml of 300 mg/l are injected. AP lateral and oblique views are taken to display the nerve roots.

Serious complications have mainly been attributed to hyperextension of the cervical spine during the examination and have been estimated at 0.023 per cent of all cervical myelograms (Robertson and Smith, 1990). Lateral C1/2 puncture may also lead to direct needle puncture injuries of the cord, but this is avoided by regular checks for CSF during needle insertion (Orrison, Sackett and Amundsen, 1983). Rarely aberrant posterior siting of the vertebral artery may lead to puncture and epidural haemorrhage (Cox, Stevens and Kendall, 1981), but this is avoided by the posterior site of needle insertion (Orrison, Sackett and Amundsen, 1983).

Anomalous dorsal curves of the vertebral artery are more frequent in patients over 50 years of age and more often involve the left artery (Cox, Stevens and Kendall, 1981).

The amount of contrast medium injected should be monitored carefully by screening during injection if complete obstruction is suspected, as excessive concentration on a section of cord may lead to cord irritation.

Hyperextension may result in a pinching effect on the cord between osteophyte or disc material and buckling of the ligamentum flavum (Breig, Turnbull and Hassler, 1966). Patients with a narrow sagittal canal, diameter below 12 mm, are particularly at risk (Epstein, Epstein and Jones, 1978). Examination of the cervical spine by magnetic resonance prior to myelography will adequately evaluate the degree of cord compression and unnecessary or dangerous cervical myelographic examination may be avoided. Prone myelography with the neck extended typically demonstrates a more severe stenosis than does MR imaging or CT myelography, which are performed in neutral or slightly flexed positions where central canal size is maximum (Sobel, Barkovich and Munderloh, 1984; Modic, Ross and Masaryk, 1989).

The hallmark of focal disc herniation at myelography is a rounded or angular indentation on the anterolateral margin of the contrast column at the disc space, with amputation of the nerve root sleeve (Figure 2.18). Osteophytes may also indent the contrast column and amputate the nerve root sleeve and the latter feature may also be seen on its own. More laterally placed osteophytes may not affect the root sleeve, which is short in the cervical spine (Fox *et al.*, 1975). CT may be performed following the planar views. Alternatively, intrathecal enhancement with dilute contrast medium inserted by lumbar puncture may also be performed and CT performed without the standard lateral and oblique views. The high spatial resolution in cross section delineates subtle intradural and extradural abnormalities and permits accurate differentiation and characterization of bone versus soft tissue lesion and direct depiction of cord and foraminal size (Figure 2.19) (Badami *et al.*, 1985; Brown *et al.*, 1988). Beam hardening artefacts may, however, diminish the quality of scans in the lower cervical region due to the shoulder (Daniels *et al.*, 1984; Brown *et al.*, 1988). The technique also uses a lower dose of intrathecal contrast medium than standard myelography, thus reducing the morbidity and side effects and may be performed on outpatients.

Myelography alone demonstrated the presence of compression of the cord or nerve roots in 95 per cent of 39 cases described by Modic *et al.* (1986), but had a lower accuracy

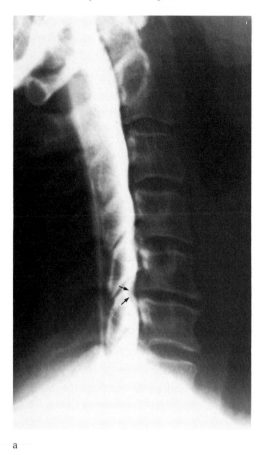
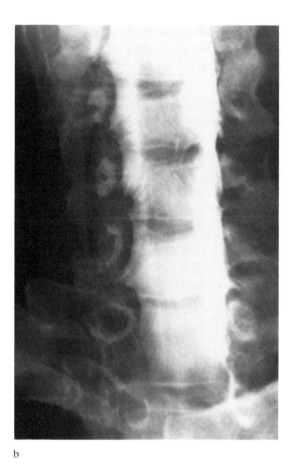

a   b

Figure 2.18. There is mild indentation of the dural sac on the lateral view at C5/6 (a), with some half shadowing is due to the posterolateral position of the prolapse. The oblique view (b) shows the amputation of the adjacent nerve root.

level of 67 per cent when the type of lesion was considered, in that herniation, bony stenosis and a combination of both were difficult to differentiate. CT myelography was superior in differentiating these features at 85 per cent, although a combination of herniation and stenosis was diagnosed purely as stenosis in three of 11 cases. The demonstration of nerve root and cord compression may be achieved without intrathecal intervention using magnetic resonance with surface coils, but in the series of Modic *et al.* (1986), this proved slightly less accurate than CT myelography, with a 92 per cent accuracy for depicting an abnormality, but only 74 per cent accuracy in differentiating osteophyte from soft tissue. Surface coil technology and imaging systems have, however, improved significantly since 1986 when this study was reported.

The main advantages of myelography lies in the dynamic nature of the contrast flow which enhances the ability to assess the degree of compression of the nerve roots in particular but also of the cord, although this is not the case if a block is present. The major advantages of magnetic resonance are its non-invasive nature, its capacity to display the foramen magnum and cervical region in its entirety and the characterization of the cord contour and delineation of signal alterations within the cord substance. It also allows easy evaluation of regions proximal to severe stenosis of block. While the study by Modic *et al.* (1986) demonstrated deficiencies in tissue characterization, recent advances with gradient echo imaging sequences have produced a 40 per cent improvement in contrast between bone and CSF in the axial and sagittal planes

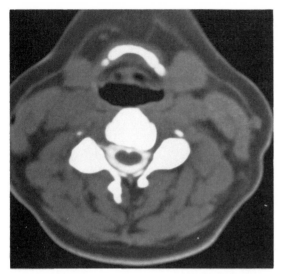

Figure 2.19. CT myelogram showing narrowing of the right intervertebral foramen by an osteophyte without cord compression.

(Kulkarni *et al.*, 1988) and disc prolapse can be differentiated from osteophyte with greater ease (see Figure 2.15). Three-dimensional imaging has also enabled thin contiguous slices with improved signal to noise ratio and special resolution to be obtained. This further improves the demonstration of low intensity spurs and high intensity herniated discs.

Delayed CT myelography 10–12 hours after intrathecal injection permits the assessment of the spinal cord damage. Accumulation of contrast may be seen in areas of cord damage, which may include focal cavities, and contrast can also be seen in syrinx of the central canal (Figure 2.20) (Dubois *et al.*, 1981; Jenkins *et al.*, 1986). However, the demonstration of intramedullary cystic changes and of syrinx formation is most easily and most effectively achieved with magnetic resonance, where the low signal area of fluid within the cord is easily demonstrated on the T1 weighted image with a corresponding high signal on T2 weighting (Yashimata *et al.*, 1990) (Figure 2.20). In the acute stage myelography may delineate evidence of disc prolapse associated with vertebral trauma but magnetic resonance is the investigation of choice as the status of the cord can be evaluated. Cord swelling and oedema appear as cord enlargement on T1 weighted images, with high signal on T2 weighted

sequences (Figure 2.21). The signal of intramedullary haemorrhage will depend on its age but early changes show as a focus of high signal intensity on T1, with low signal on T2 (Flaunders *et al.*, 1990). Herniation of the intervertebral disc in association with trauma is also easily visualized with MR and an incidence of 47 per cent has been reported in studies of unstable injuries of the cervical spine (Pratt, Green and Spengler, 1990).

Provocative radiology

The failure of imaging clearly to differentiate those pathological changes which are due to the ageing process from those that are a source of clinical symptoms has led to the development of investigations which, while demonstrating anatomical changes, also provide crucial information by their reproduction or abolition of symptoms during the procedure. Such investigations require specialist skills and it is important that they are undertaken by the radiologist only after detailed consultation with the surgeon and when a precise course of action for the patient has been decided.

Cervical discography

This investigation is now performed infrequently and is only of value in those cases of cervical pain whose symptoms are severe enough to warrant surgical intervention. It is not indicated if the symptoms, signs or EMG studies indicate that a radiculopathy is present. In such cases cervical myelography, CT myelography or MR are the investigations of choice.

If the neck pain is sclerotomal, however, and it is not clear from which level the pain is originating, then discography is of value. The disc is approached from the anterolateral aspect medial to the carotid artery and lateral to the pharynx. A 21 gauge needle is placed against the anterolateral aspect of the annulus after local infiltration of anaesthetic. A 26 gauge needle is passed through the 21 gauge and into the centre of the nucleus. The position of the needle tip is confirmed by screening in the AP and lateral planes. Water soluble non-ionic contrast medium is then injected into the nucleus. A normal disc will not accept more

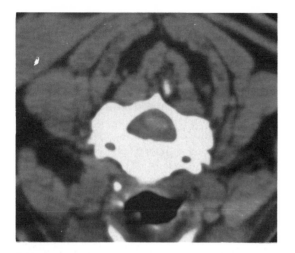

a

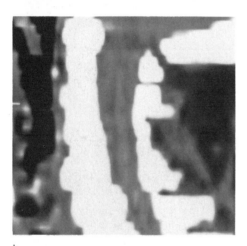

b

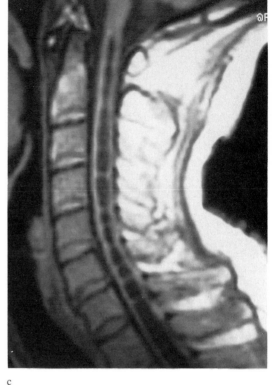

c

Figure 2.20. Post-traumatic syrinx. The CT myelogram with delayed imaging shows dilute contrast in the distended central canal on (a) the axial scan and (b) the sagittal reconstruction. (c) A T1 weighted MR scan also shows clearly the low signal of the dilated canal within the cord substance.

than 0.2 ml of contrast medium and will appear as a central opacity (Figure 2.22). However, contrast commonly leaks through posterolateral clefts into the neurocentral joints in the third decade onwards and this is a normal feature for this age group (Holt, 1964). Contrast may, however, pass through a tear in the posterior annulus centrally and a localized bulge can be seen extending beyond the posterior wall of the vertebral bodies and this type of lesion is more likely to be of symptomatic significance.

Any pain induced during the injection of contrast is recorded and the distribution, character and intensity of the pain compared with the patient's normal symptoms. Following the stimulation of pain by contrast, a small quantity of local anaesthetic, usually 0.1–0.2

ml, may be injected into the disc to assess any reduction in pain. Care must be taken not to use too much local anaesthetic if there is considerable epidural leakage through the posterior annulus as this may block a pain response from a subsequent disc injection. It is very unusual to inject more than three discs and it may be valuable to undertake the individual levels on different days if significant symptoms are induced.

The accuracy of cervical discography is difficult to assess. There is more overlap of the sclerotomal zones in the cervical spine compared with the lumbar spine, but Simmons and Segil (1975) found a good correlation between the demonstration of symptoms and the result of subsequent surgery to 91 per cent

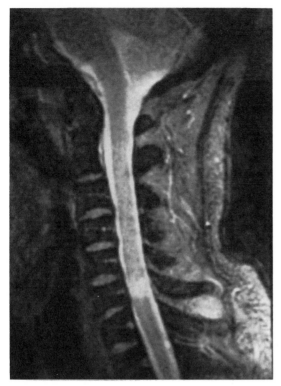

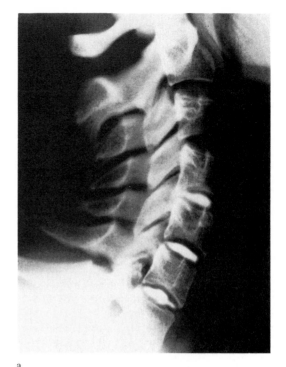

a

Figure 2.21. Hyperflexion injury. The T2 weighted MR scan shows increased signal in the cord due to oedema. There is also increase in signal in the interspinous ligament at the same level.

of patients, while other authors suggest that 70 per cent have proved to have a good result following demonstration of a symptomatic level (Whitecloud and Seago, 1987). The investigation, however, is not without its detractors (Klafta and Collis, 1969; Meriam and Stockdale, 1983) who conclude that it is non-specific in both anatomical demonstration and symptom reproduction. Cervical discography is not without hazard as subsequent disc infection may occur and the incidence appears to be higher than the 0.4 per cent quoted for lumbar discography (Fraser, Osti and Vernon-Roberts, 1989). The investigation is performed under a single prophylactic systemic injection of antibiotics but the prophylactic value of this is not, as yet, proven in cervical discography. Extra care should also be taken if previous cervical surgery has been performed, due to the pharynx becoming adherent to the prevertebral fascia.

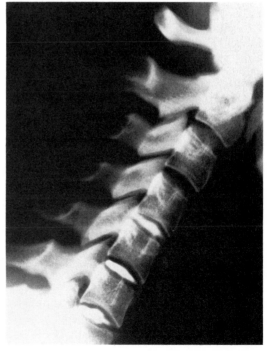

b

Figure 2.22. Cervical discograms. The C4/5 shows a small cleft in the posterior annulus, which is accentuated by extension. The C5/6 and 6/7 levels are normal.

Cervical facet injections

The cervical facet joints may also be a cause of neck pain and their direct investigation has been substantially neglected. The features of degeneration have already been recorded and the fact that degeneration is a regular feature in the older subject makes it impossible to differentiate the symptomatic and incidental changes by plain films, MR or CT. Local anaesthetic blocks of the medial branches of the cervical dorsal rami have therefore been advocated as a method of investigation of patients with chronic neck pain. The 22 gauge needle is placed in the medial branches of the cervical dorsal rami from a posterolateral approach under screen control and local anaesthetic is injected. Bogduk and Marsland (1988) found 17 out of 24 cases of chronic neck pain had complete relief, which was confirmed on repeat injections and seven also had pain relief from injections into the facet joints. No controls, however, were included in this series and no attempt was made to categorize the type of pain or to inject water into the symptomatic group as a comparative study.

Asymptomatic subjects have been studied to assess the distribution of pain referral. The facet joints were distended with contrast medium and the areas of pain induced from different facet levels were mapped out. Using these pain distribution patterns in symptomatic patients anaesthetic blocks of the related facet joints were undertaken and a successful result was achieved in nine out of 10 patients at the predicted level (Aprill, Dwyer and Bogduk, 1990).

However, the value of facet injections in the cervical spine requires considerable further evaluation before this technique should be used for routine use.

Vertebral angiography

Abnormalities in the cervical spine may produce clinical symptoms removed from its immediate locality. This is particularly the case with involvement of the vertebral arteries during their passage through the cervical spine. The incidence of vertebral artery compression by osteophytes, facet hypertrophy or spondylolisthesis, due to degeneration

or destruction is not clear but it is a well recognized cause of lateral medullary syndrome and less florid lesions.

The flow through the vertebral artery can be assessed by vertebral angiography, which is performed by catheterization of the origin of the vertebral artery via a puncture in the femoral artery. Injection of contrast into the subclavian artery may produce sufficient opacification of the vertebral artery and may be of value in the older patient, where direct vertebral injection is contraindicated. Anteroposterior and lateral views of the opacified artery are taken during the injection of a small quantity of contrast medium.

Vertebral artery evaluation may also be achieved with digital subtraction angiography following intravenous or intradural injection of contrast. This is now an effective procedure and is the investigation of choice in the older patient.

Conclusion

There is now a variety of investigative procedures for the cervical spine and the choice of the most appropriate technique is in part dependent on the clinical presentation. Plain radiographs remain essential and can provide much basic information and, supplemented by magnetic resonance imaging, most conditions can be fully assessed. CT remains valuable if bone lesions are present and invasive procedures may be required for final evaluation prior to surgery. In all circumstances close cooperation between clinician and radiologist is essential for a successful outcome.

References

Aprill, C., Dwyer, A. and Bogduk, N. (1990) Cervical zygapophyseal joint pain patterns (II). A clinical evaluation. *Spine*, **15**, 458–461.

Badami, J.P., Norman, D., Barbara, N.M., Caum, C.E., Weinstein, P.R. and Sobel, D.F. (1985) Metrizamide CT myelography and radiculography correlation with conventional myelography and surgical findings. *American Journal of Neuroradiology*, **6**, 59–64.

Boden, S.C., McCowin, P.R., Davis, D.O., Dina, T.S., Mark, A.S. and Wiesel, S. (1990) Abnormal magnetic resonance scans of the cervical spine in asymptomatic subjects. *Journal of Bone and Joint Surgery*, **72A**, 1178–1184.

Bogduk, N. and Marsland, A. (1988). The cervical zygapophyseal joints as a source of neck pain. *Spine*, **13**, 610–617.

Brain, W.R. (1962) Some unresolved problems of cervical spondylosis. *British Medical Journal*, **1**, 771–777.

Breig, A., Turnbull, I. and Hassler, O. (1966) Effects of mechanical stresses on the spinal cord in cervical spondylosis. *Journal of Neurosurgery*, **25(1)**, 45–56.

Brown, B.M., Schwartz, R.H., Frank, E. and Blank, N.K. (1988). Preoperative evaluation of cervical radiculopathy and myelography by surface coil MR imaging. *American Journal of Roentgenology*, **151**, 1205–1212.

Bundschuh, C., Modic, M.T., Kearney, F., Norris, R. and Deal, C. (1988) Rheumatoid arthritis of the cervical spine: surface coil MR imaging. *American Journal of Roentgenology*, **151**, 181–188.

Burrows, E.H. (1963) Sagittal diameter of the spinal cord in cervical spondylosis. *Clinical Radiology*, **14**, 77–83.

Chamberlain, W.E. (1939) Basilar impression. *Yale Journal of Biological Medicine*, **11**, 487–488.

Cox, T.C.S., Stevens, J.M. and Kendall, B.E. (1981) Vascular anatomy in the sub-occipital region and lateral cervical puncture. *British Journal of Radiology*, **54**, 572–575.

Daniels, D.L., Grogan, J.P., Johansen, J.G., Meyer, C.A., Williams, A.L. and Haughton, I.M. (1984) Cervical radiculography: computed tomography and myelography compared. *Radiology*, **151**, 109–113.

Dubois, P.J., Drayer, B.P., Sage, M., Osborne, D. and Heinz, M.R. (1981) Intramedullary penetrance of metrizamide in the dog spinal cord. *American Journal of Neuroradiology*, **2**, 313–317.

Epstein, B.S., Epstein, J.A. and Jones, M.D. (1978) Anatomicro-radiological correlations in cervical discal disease and stenosis. *Clinical Neurosurgery*, **25**, 148–173.

Flaunders, A.E., Shaefer, S.M., Doan, H.T., Miskkin, M.M., Gonzales, C.F. and Northrup, B.E. (1990) Acute cervical spine trauma in correlation of MR imaging findings with degree of neurological deficit. *Radiology*, **177**, 25–33.

Fletcher, G., Haughton, V.M., Ho, K.S. and Yu, S. (1990) Age related changes in cervical facet joint studies with cryomicrotomy MR and CT. *American Journal of Roentgenology*, **154**, 817–820.

Fox, A.T., Lin, J.P., Pinto, R.S. and Krichelf, I.T. (1975) Myelographic cervical nerve root deformities. *Radiology*, **116**, 355–361.

Fraser, R.D., Osti, O.L. and Vernon-Roberts, B. (1989) Iatogenic discitis: the role of intravenous antibiotics in prevention and treatment. *Spine*, **14**, 1025–1032.

Jenkins, J.R., Bashir, R., Al Mefty, O., Al-Kawi, M.Z. and Fox, J.L. (1986) Cystic necrosis of the spinal cord in compressive cervical myelopathy demonstration by iopamidol CT myelography. *American Journal of Neuroradiology*, **7**, 693–701.

Hink, V.C., Hopkins, C.E. and Savara, B.S. (1961) Diagnostic criteria of basilar impression. *Radiology*, **76**, 572–576.

Holt, E.P. (1964) Fallacy of cervical discography: report of 50 cases in normal subjects. *Journal of American Medical Association*, **188**, 799–801.

Klafta, L.A. and Collis, J.S. (1969) An analysis of cervical discography with surgical verifications. *Journal of Neurosurgery*, **30**, 38–41.

Kulkarni, M.V., Narayana, P.A., McArdle, C.B., Yeakley, J.W., Campagna, N.F. and Wehrli, F.W. (1988) Cervical spine MR imaging using multislice gradient echo imaging: comparison with cardiac gated spin echo. *Magnetic Resonance Imaging*, **6**, 517–526.

McCall, I.W., Park, W.M., McSweeney, T. (1973) The radiological demonstration of lower cervical injury. *Clinical Radiology*, **34**, 235–240.

McGregor, M. (1948) Measurements in diagnosis of basilar impression. *British Journal of Radiology*, **21**, 171–173.

Merkel, K.D., Fitzgerald, R.H. Jr and Brown, M.L. (1984) Scintigraphic evaluation in musculo-skeletal sepsis. *Orthopaedic Clinics of North America*, **15(3)**, 401–416.

Meriam, W.F. and Stockdale, H.R. (1983) Is cervical discography of any value? *European Journal of Radiology*, **3**, 138–141.

Modic, M.T., Masaryk, T.J., Mulopulos, G.P., Bundschuk, C., Han, J.S. and Bohlman, H. (1986) Cervical radiculopathy: prospective evaluation with surface coil MR imaging; CT with metrizamide and metrizamide myelography. *Radiology*, **161**, 753–759.

Modic, M.T., Ross, J.S. and Masaryk, T.J. (1989) Imaging of degenerative disease of the cervical spine. *Clinical Orthopaedics*, **239**, 109–120.

National Radiation Protection Board (1990) Patient dose reduction in diagnostic radiology, **1**(3) 17.

Orrison, W.W., Sackett, J.F. and Amundsen, P. (1983) Lateral C1–2 puncture for cervical myelography 11. Recognition of improper injection of contrast material. *Radiology*, **146**, 395–400.

Patton, D.D. and Woolfenden, J.M. (1977) Radionucleide bone scanning in diseases of the spine. *Radiologic Clinics of North America*, **15**, 177–201.

Petterson, H., Larsson, E.M., Holtas, S. *et al.* (1988) MR imaging of the cervical spine in rheumatoid arthritis. *American Journal of Neuroradiology*, **9**, 573–577.

Pratt, E.S., Green, D.A. and Spengler, D.M. (1990) Herniated intervertebral discs associated with unstable injuries. *Spine*, **15**, 662–666.

Robertson, H.J. and Smith, R.D. (1990) Cervical myelography: survey of modes of practice and major complications. *Radiology*, **174**, 79–83.

Simmons, E.H. and Segil, C.M. (1975) An evaluation of discography in the localisation of symptomatic levels in discogenic disease of the spine. *Clinical Orthopaedics and Related Research*, **108**, 59–69.

Sobel, D.F., Barkovich, A.J. and Munderloh, S.H. (1984) Metrizamide myelography and postmyelographic computed tomography comparative adequacy in cervical spine. *American Journal of Neuroradiology*, **5**, 385–390.

Szypryt, E.P., Hardy, J.G., Hinton, C.E., Worthington, B.S. and Mulholland, R.C. (1988) A comparison between magnetic resonance imaging and scintigraphic bone imaging in the diagnosis of disc space infection in an animal model. *Spine*, **13**, 1042–1048.

Tchang, S.P.K. (1974) The cervical spino-laminar line. *Journal of Association of Canadian Radiologists*, **25**, 224–226.

Wakeley, C.J., Cassar-Pullicino, V.N. and McCall, I.W. (1991) Case of the month: not so pseudo. *British Journal of Radiology*, **64**, 375–376.

Whitecloud, T.S. and Seago, R.A. (1987) Cervical discogenic syndrome. Result of operative intervention in patients with positive discography. *Spine*, **12**, 313–316.

Yashimata, Y., Takahashi, M., Matsumo, Y. *et al.* (1990) Chronic injuries of the spinal cord. Assessment MR imaging. *Radiology*, **175**, 849–854.

3 Congenital malformations and deformities of the cervical spine

*'Deep in the cavern of the infants breast
the father's nature lurks and lives anew.'*

Horace (Odes 4)

Congenital anomalies of the cervical spine vary from gross failures of development that are incompatible with life to anomalies that are discovered by chance radiography and are of no significance. They can occur singly, be multiple within the cervical spine or be but one feature of multiple congenital deformities affecting other systems. When this last occurs, the cervical anomaly may have the solitary significance of adding another name to an already polyeponymic recondite syndrome.

Classification of cervical anomalies is best done on anatomical grounds, understanding that most anomalies result from failure of fusion, or failure of segmentation, of developmental components. Congenital anomalies become clinically significant if they compromise the spinal cord or threaten the stability of the cervical spine.

Development of the cervical spine

The vertebral column passes through four stages of development (Figure 3.1). The unsegmented notochord extends towards the head and becomes incorporated into the sphenoid. Tissue is laid down to form a mesenchymal column, segmented into 35 units. These units become the protovertebrae, divided into equal cephalic and caudal parts by a transient linear gap, the sclerotomic fissure. From the caudal half a dorsal extension outlines the neural arch and another extension grows laterally between corresponding myotomes.

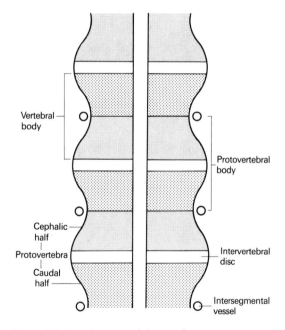

Figure 3.1. Development of the vertebrae.

As these extensions appear the caudal part of each protovertebral segment fuses with the cephalic part of the adjacent segment forming an intersegmental mesodermal centrum. The tissues adjacent to the sclerotomic fissure condense to form the perichordal disc, the future annulus of the intervertebral disc. The notochord atrophies except in the area of the perichordal disc where it persists as the nucleus pulposus until its ultimate disappearance in the second decade of life.

The third stage is chondrification of the mesodermal vertebrae. Two centres fuse in the sixth week to form a cartilaginous centrum, and each half of the neural arch chondrifies from a centre which rapidly fuses with the centrum to form the pedicle, and extends dorsally as a cartilaginous lamina to meet its fellow in the third month. The transverse processes extend laterally in continuity with the neural arch, but the costal processes chondrify separately and become the anterior arch of the foramen transversarium. In the first three vertebrae the costal elements are united across the front of the centrum by the hypochondral bow. This structure persists only in the atlas as its anterior arch; the centrum of the atlas joins the axis as the odontoid process.

Ossification begins towards the end of the second month of intrauterine life. The primary centres appear first at the roots of the transverse processes and ossification spreads into the pedicles and laminae.

The centrum ossifies from one, sometimes two, centres dorsal to the notochord. When two such centres fail to fuse, a hemivertebra is formed. Until the second year of life the centrum is connected to each vertebral arch by a synchondrosis. The anterior part of the arch becomes the neurocentral lip of the mature vertebra.

Six secondary centres appear at puberty. These are two annular circumferential epiphyseal discs above and below the body, two secondary centres at the tip of the spinous process and two more at the tips of the transverse processes. Occasionally these secondary centres do not fuse with the primary centres at the end of skeletal growth.

The atlas and axis ossify differently.

The atlas ossifies from three centres. Those of the two lateral masses appear in the seventh intrauterine week and extend backwards into the posterior arch to unite in the fourth year. The centre for the anterior arch does not appear until the end of the first year of life. Union with the lateral masses occurs at about 6 years. Occasionally this centre does not appear and ossification occurs by forward extension of the two lateral centres.

The centrum and arches of the axis are formed from three or four primary centres as in a typical vertebra. The odontoid represents the centrum of the atlas. Two primary centres, one either side of the midline appear in early intrauterine life and are fused together by birth. At birth the space between 'atlas' and 'axis' is formed by a synchondrosis. This lies below the level of the superior facets of the atlas, lower than the base of the mature odontoid process. The body and the odontoid fuse by 6 years. If union does not occur the appearances may be misinterpreted as a fracture or vice versa. Fractures through the base of the odontoid, however, occur at the level of the articular facets (Blockley and Purser, 1956; Fielding, 1965; Freiberger, Wilson and Nicholas, 1965; Seimon, 1977). This pattern of ossification is reflected in the blood supply of the odontoid. There is a vascular watershed between the odontoid and the body of the axis, between branches of the vertebral and carotid systems. This is thought to be a contributory factor in non-union of odontoid fractures (Schiff and Parke, 1972).

A secondary centre appears above the cleft tip of the process in the second year and unites at puberty. This represents the 'pro-atlas', the cranial half of the first cervical protovertebra. The pro-atlas is a normal anatomical structure in reptiles. In man it may persist ununited as the ossiculum terminale, attached to the rest of the odontoid by cartilage. It has been reported as a cause of atlanto-axial instability (Sherk and Nicholson, 1969; Finerman, Sakai and Weingarten, 1976). In radiographs of infants the unossified tip of the odontoid may be misinterpreted by the unwary as odontoid hypoplasia or atlanto-axial subluxation.

The costal elements of the seventh cervical vertebra may persist as cervical ribs. They can be identified by their downwards projection.

Classification of bony anomalies of the cervical spine

Tidy classification is difficult because many separate anomalies can coexist. They may be incidental radiographic findings, and remain so unless degenerative changes in later life reduce the margin of safety in a vulnerable canal.

The bony anomalies may be grouped, for ease of description, as:

1 Anomalies of the craniovertebral junction.
2 Anomalies causing atlanto-axial instability.
3 Anomalies of the lower cervical spine.

The practical questions for the practising surgeon are:

1 Is the lesion unstable?
2 Is there a risk of neurological damage?
3 Is there an associated anomaly of the brain-stem or cord?

1 Anomalies of the craniovertebral junction

There is a variety of conditions, congenital and acquired, where the anatomical relations between the base of the skull and the upper two cervical vertebrae are disturbed. It is important to be clear what is meant by the different terms used to describe these appearances.

Basilar coarctation describes congenital invagination of the odontoid into the foramen magnum.

Basilar impression describes acquired invagination of the odontoid into the foramen magnum.

Platybasia is an anthropometric term describing flattening of the base of the skull. The angle subtended by the clivus and episthion should not be more than 130°.

The various diagnostic lines that can be drawn on standard radiographs are described in Chapter 8. They are difficult to draw on films of the infantile skeleton and reliance should be on computed tomographic (CT) scanning or magnetic resonance imaging (MRI).

Basilar coarctation

Congenital malformation of the foramen magnum allows the tip of the odontoid to be higher than normal, even to the point of compromising the brainstem. Other skeletal anomalies may coexist, but the peculiar association of basilar coarctation is with the Arnold–Chiari phenomen. This malformation consists of caudal prolapse of the tonsils of the cerebellum. There may be hydrocephalus and there is a high association with lumbar myelomeningocele. The vertebral arteries are often compromised and the ischaemia which follows may be the cause of the often associated syringomyelia (Figure 3.2) (Chiari, 1891; Arnold, 1903; Michie and Clark, 1968).

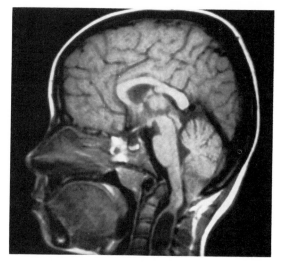

Figure 3.2. Arnold–Chiari phenomenon with syringomyelia. (Mr Gordon Finlay's case.)

Some degree of cerebellar tonsillar prolapse may not produce symptoms during life or until additional compression is created by trauma or degeneration (Taylor and Byrnes, 1974). Basilar coarctation in itself may also not be a cause of symptoms until adolescence, adulthood or even throughout life. Clinical symptoms and signs can be varied and complex.

The long tracts of the brainstem, the tonsils of the cerebellum and the lower cranial nerves may all, or separately, be compressed. Vertebral artery compression can produce varying degrees of the lateral medullary syndrome, ranging from transient loss of consciousness to the fully established Wallenberg syndrome (Wallenberg, 1897; Klein, Snyder and Schwartz, 1976; and see Chapter 7). The neurological symptoms of limb pain, ataxia and sensory disturbances may bring the patient to the orthopaedic clinic (Taylor and Byrnes, 1974).

The mechanical problems of management are of stenosis of the foramen magnum, or craniovertebral instability. The two may exist together, the instability causing intermittent stenosis. The surgical management of these lesions belongs to the neurosurgeon, but the orthopaedic surgeon may be called on to treat the instability which follows the decompression of the neurosurgical procedure (Hamblen, 1967).

The extension of internal fixation devices, such as the Ransford loop, to the skull, has allowed extensive anterior or posterior decompression operations free of anxiety about postoperative instability (Crockard and Ransford, 1985)

Occipitalization of the atlas

Congenital fusion of the atlas to the skull is usually ascribed to a failure of segmentation of the pro-atlas. However, the element most often fused to the occiput is the anterior arch of the atlas, derived from the hypochordal bow (Hadley, 1946). The assimilation usually includes the lateral masses and the atlanto-occipital joints. The posterior arch is sometimes discrete, but hypoplastic, compressing the dura and the cord. Fusion of the anterior arch to the occiput can displace the odontoid backwards, and the assimilation reduces the height of the interval between atlas and skull. If the tip of the odontoid projects into the foramen magnum symptoms of brainstem compression are likely. If the tip lies below the level of the foramen symptoms are unlikely.

In a majority of patients with occipitalization of the atlas, there is also fusion between C2 and C3. The atlanto-axial joint is then the only articulation between the skull and the lower cervical spine. The stress on this joint is likely to produce instability and neural compromise even in the absence of an abnormally placed odontoid (McRae, 1953; Torklus and Giehle, 1972).

Other congenital anomalies are associated. There may be kyphosis or scoliosis. Patients with occipitalization look like patients affected by the Klippel-Feil syndrome in that they have a short, stiff neck and torticollis (McRae, 1953). Facial malformations, hypospadias and malformations of the genito-urinary tract, pes cavus and syndactly have been reported (Spillane, Pallis and Jones, 1957). The surgeon must remember that when a congenital cervical anomaly is found he or she should look for defects elsewhere.

The onset of a clinical picture is associated with trauma, or delayed into adult life. Anterior compression of the medulla by an abnormal odontoid peg will produce long tract signs of spasticity (Bharucha and Dastur, 1964). The hypoplastic posterior arch of the atlas, if present, may indent the cord and produce posterior column signs with loss of proprioception. The immediate cause of this presentation is atlanto-axial instability, either abruptly following injury, or progressively with the cumulative effects of intermittent compression. With advancing age, connective tissue loses its elasticity, joints become stiffer so that the long lever of the lower cervical spine becomes more rigid and arteries become sclerotic.

If symptoms and signs appear suddenly after injury, simple protection of the neck with a collar may allow resolution. If neurological deterioration continues, operative decompression is necessary. Operations on this condition are dangerous. Anterior decompression by the transoral route, using microsurgical techniques, immediately followed by posterior occipitocervical fixation, is the most effective and safest procedure (Crockard and Ransford, 1985).

2 Anomalies causing atlanto-axial instability

A number of anomalies associated with the odontoid have in common atlanto-axial instability which can cause neurological damage from compression of the spinal cord.

The stability of the atlanto-axial joint depends on the integrity of the odontoid process, the transverse ligament of the atlas and the alar ligaments (see Chapter 1). If these ligaments are deficient and the odontoid is intact the cord is at risk of being compressed when the head and neck are flexed. If the odontoid is deficient the cord is vulnerable during flexion and extension.

Anomalies of the odontoid process

The apex of the odontoid ossifies from a secondary centre appearing in the second year of life. If it does not unite by bone with the two primary centres the persistent bony nodule is the ossiculum terminale. Cases have been reported where the anomaly has been associated with atlanto-axial dislocation (Sherk and Nicholson, 1969; Finerman, Sakai and Weingarten, 1976). The delayed appearance of the secondary ossification centre must be remembered when interpreting radiographs of infants as the anterior arch of the atlas will seem to lie above the tip of the odontoid. When the ossiculum is present it must be differentiated from os odontoideum.

Os odontoideum is a round or oval ossicle separated from a hypoplastic odontoid base. It is considerably larger than an ossiculum terminale and has a cortical circumference. It may be fused with the occiput. It is held, with some justification, that the os odontoideum represents an ununited fracture of the base of the odontoid and is not a congenital anomaly. Much has been written in support of either view (Gillman, 1959; Gwinn and Smith, 1962; Fielding, 1965; Torklus and Gehle, 1972; Fielding and Griffin, 1974; Seimon, 1977; Fielding, Hensinger and Hawkins, 1980).

The congenital theory postulates either a failure of fusion of the apical centre to the primary centres of ossification or a failure of the odontoid to fuse to the body of the axis. As we have seen, an os odontoideum is bigger than and has a different appearance from an ossiculum terminale. We have also seen how the synchondrosis between the odontoid and the body of the axis lies below the level of the superior articular facets, so that failure of bony fusion here could not result in a hypoplastic base. Unlike other cervical anomalies, the association of other cranioverterbral anomalies with os odontoideum is very low.

Fielding postulates the following sequence of events. An unrecognized fracture of the base of the odontoid occurs. The vascular watershed at the base of the process encourages non-union of the fracture. The alar ligaments, attached to the tip of the odontoid, contract with time and pull the fragment upwards unopposed by any bony healing. The smooth cortical circumference is due to established pseudo-arthrosis. Support for this hypothesis is derived from the natural history of a number of cases of united fractures of the base of the odontoid (Fielding, Hensinger and Hawkins, 1980).

The same arguments are advanced to explain odontoid hypoplasia. Avascular necrosis of the odontoid has been observed following prolonged halopelvic traction (Tredwell and O'Brien, 1975). Hypoplasia and os odontoideum have also been reported after pyogenic osteomyelitis (Freiberger, Wilson and Nicholas, 1965; Ahlback and Collert, 1970). However, true congenital hypoplasia

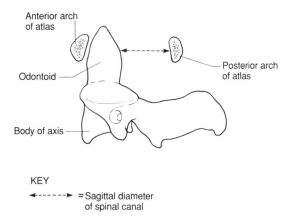

Figure 3.3. Atlanto-axial stability.

has been described (Shepard, 1966; Michaels, Provost and Croug, 1989). Congenital aplasia, complete absence of the odontoid, can only be diagnosed when the body of the axis does not project above the level of the superior articular surfaces.

Patients with atlanto-axial instability due to odontoid anomalies will present with symptoms and signs ranging from discomfort in the neck to a progressive tetraparesia. Vertigo and syncope may be due to constriction of the vertebral arteries (McKeever, 1968) and there may be involvement of the cranial nerves (Minderhoud, Brakman and Penning, 1969).

The anomaly will be apparent on standard radiographs but flexion/extension studies will reveal the degree of atlanto-axial instability. MRI, with its ability to demonstrate the degree of compromise of the cord is the investigation of first choice.

The management of these patients is difficult. If there is a progressive neurological defect the unstable segment must be fused. Doubt arises in the management of those patients whose symptoms are minimal, and those who are without symptoms, and whose anomaly is found on chance radiography. The case against prophylactic fusion is that the operation is dangerous and that patients with such anomalies are not at risk if they avoid athletic activities (Gillman, 1959; Garber, 1964; Shepard, 1966; Fielding, Hensinger and Hawkins, 1980). They remain vulnerable to accidental trauma, however, and it is cruel to restrict sporting activities when Western society places such high value on athletic ability.

If possible, any atlanto-axial displacement should be first reduced by positioning of the head, or gentle traction. If there has been a neurological defect there should then be a waiting period of 10–14 days before operation so that the irritated cord can settle. The operation of choice is posterior occipitocervical fusion, with internal fixation permitting early postoperative mobility. If the displacement cannot be reduced the choice lies between fusion in situ, and transoral decompression combined with occipitocervical fixation (Crockard and Ransford, 1985). An option which is *not* open is to attempt a blind reduction on the operating table (Nicholson and Sherk, 1968; Sinto and Pandya, 1968).

The association of os odontoideum with ununited fractures of the odontoid should not be advanced as a reason for internal fixation of odontoid fractures. The association of non-union is with traction, not with splintage. If non-union does occur, and is associated with instability, posterior atlanto-axial fixation and fusion is a much safer operation.

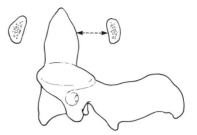

Figure 3.4. Atlanto-axial instability. Odontoid intact.

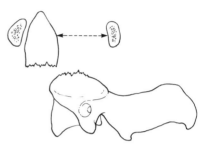

Figure 3.5. Atlanto-axial instability. Odontoid mobile. Cruciate ligament intact.

Spondyolysis and spondylolisthesis

Failure of fusion between the neural arch and the centrum is not usually associated with atlanto-axial instability. It has been described in association with odontoid aplasia (Jeffreys, 1980).

Congenital laxity of the cruciate ligament

This diagnosis can only be made when there is atlanto-axial instability, and bony anomalies, injury, infection and rheumatoid disease have been excluded as responsible factors.

Craniovertebral anomalies in cervical dysplasia (Figures 3.3, 3.4 and 3.5)

Many children suffering from skeletal dysplasia have anomalies of the craniovertebral area and most of these anomalies are of the odontoid. All children with Morquio's disease have the malformation. The incidence of bony anomaly is less than that of atlanto-axial instability and neurological damage. Flexion and extension radiographs, or cine radiography of active, never passive, movement should be part of the routine screening of these children as soon as they can cooperate (Wynne-Davies *et al.*, 1989).

The soft tissues are also faulty in Morquio's disease and atlanto-axial displacement is inevitable. The onset of symptoms and signs is insidious and present as fatigue, or complaints of tingling in the extremities. Assessment is difficult because of the joint laxity characteristic of the condition. The head and neck may be held extended because 'it feels safe'. Long tract signs and ordinary retention appear late. Parents must be vigilant for early symptoms. Quarterly neurological examination is advised by the Skeletal Advisory Group (Wynne-Davies *et al.*, 1989).

Atlanto-axial fusion should be deferred as long as possible. Even at the age of seven or eight the operation field is no more than two centimetres square. There is much cartilage and it is not easy to obtain bony fusion (Lloyd Roberts, 1971). The surgical skill that can achieve success in these circumstances is rare and precious.

Atlanto-axial instability in Down's syndrome
(Figures 3.6 and 3.7)

One in five patients affected by Down's syndrome has atlanto-axial instability from attenuated or absent transverse ligaments. Only the intact alar ligaments stabilize the odontoid (Burke, French and Roberts, 1985). Yet no more than 37 cases of neurological damage had been reported by 1988 (Davidson, 1988). Four of these cases presented after athletic injury and had experienced no premonitory symptoms. Two were injured on a trampoline. All the others developed some neurological symptoms at least 4 weeks before signs appeared. There were five deaths in the series, two being sudden.

The radiographic finding of atlanto-axial displacement does not necessarily mean there is instability. Patients can become unstable from a demonstrated stability, but others can become stable after having been shown to be unstable. The natural history is unpredictable, but there does appear to be an association with upper respiratory infection.

Activities such as horse riding, cycling and gymnastics are dangerous for patients with Down's syndrome (American Academy Pediatric Committee on Sports Medicine, 1984; Acheson, 1986). Children who are eager to take part in athletics should be screened and

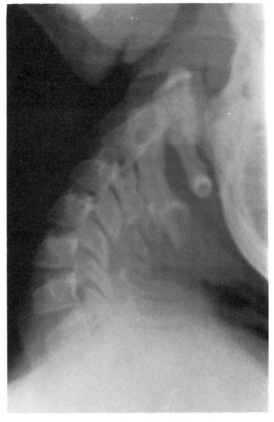

Figure 3.6. Atlanto-axial instability in Down's syndrome. Lateral view in extension.

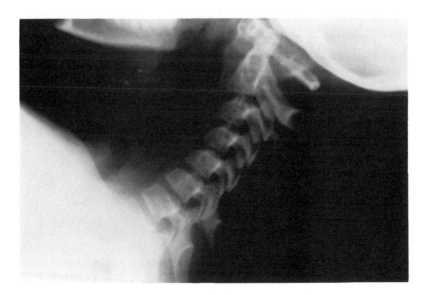

Figure 3.7. Atlanto-axial instability in Down's syndrome. Lateral view in flexion. (Mr G.A. Evans' case.)

their parents warned of the risks. The consensus is that prophylactic fusion of atlas and axis is not justified. If any child with Down's syndrome requires a general anaesthetic, the stability or otherwise of the atlanto-axial joints must be assessed.

3 Anomalies of the lower cervical spine

Congenital cervical fusion – the Klippel–Feil syndrome (Figures 3.8–3.12)

In 1912 Klippel and Feil reported on the post-mortem findings in a 46-year-old tailor who had died of pneumonia (Klippel and Feil, 1912). In life he had been known to have a short, stiff neck and a low posterior hairline. At post-mortem they found his cervical vertebrae fused into one short column, in which they could identify four vertebrae. The base of the skull approximated to the shoulders. Their eponymous association with the condition was ensured by their reporting the same case in four different journals in the same year (*Bulletin Société Anthropologie*, *Presse Medicale*, *Bulletin Société Anatomie* and the *Nouvelle Icongraphie de la Salpetrière*). So successful were they that the name has become attached to any anomaly that includes lower cervical synostosis. Feil later collected a total of fourteen cases and divided the syndrome into three types (Feil, 1919).

> *Type I* is the original syndrome of cervical synostosis with the clinical triad of a short, stiff neck and a low posterior hairline.
> *Type II* includes cervical synostosis of two or more vertebrae but without the clinical features of type I.
> *Type III* – extensive spinal synostosis involving the cervical, thoracic and lumbar spines.

The term Klippel-Feil syndrome is now used loosely to describe all variations of lower cervical synostosis. Radiographs show that the 'ghosts' of the disc spaces in congenital synostosis are in the situation which would be occupied by normal discs, so any teratogenic effect has occurred after segmentation of the protovertebrae, probably in the eighth week. It is possible that the isolated two segment fusions seen in type II are specific genetic abnormalities. The very high incidence of associated multisystem anomalies suggests that

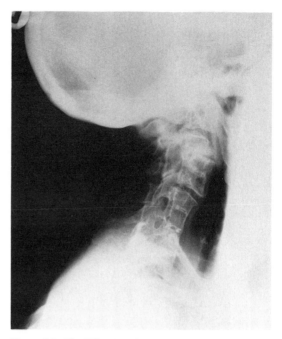

Figure 3.8. The Klippel–Feil syndrome. Type I.

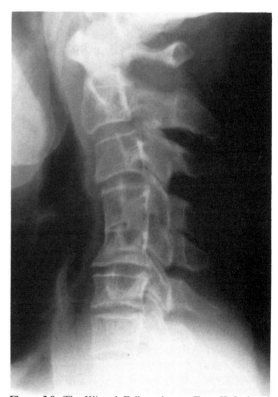

Figure 3.9. The Klippel–Feil syndrome. Type II. Isolated block vertebrae.

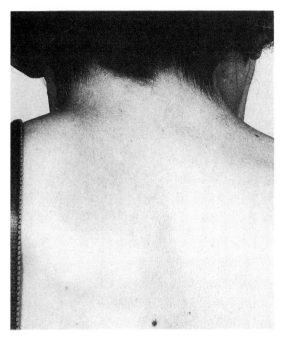

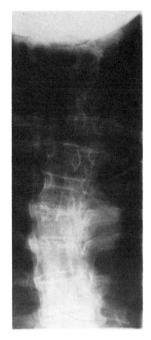

Figure 3.11. Thoracic scoliosis in Klippel–Feil syndrome.

Figure 3.10. Low hairline in Klippel–Feil syndrome.

more general, probably multifactorial, causes operate (Gunderson *et al.*, 1967). The syndrome has been called 'a constellation of associated anomalies' (Hensinger, Lang and McEwan, 1974).

Patients with type II syndromes do not present clinically unless they have an injury, or the anomaly is revealed when they present with degenerative cervical disease in middle age. Congenital synostosis can be recognized by the narrow sagittal width of the vertebral body at the level of the obliterated disc; the 'wasp waisted fusion'. The radiographic appearances of the classical syndrome are unmistakable. They may be difficult to demonstrate in the infant but bony fusion of the posterior elements will be apparent when endplate ossification of the body is incomplete.

The sagittal width of the spinal canal in the fused segments is usually normal or greater than normal. Cases have been reported of myelopathy due to spinal stenosis associated with the Klippel–Feil syndrome (Lee and Weiss, 1981; Prosick *et al.*, 1985). The intervertebral foramina in the fused segments are smaller and rounder than usual. Compression neuropathy of nerve roots in these small foramina have been reported (Okada *et al.*, 1980).

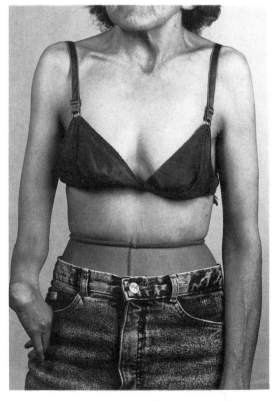

Figure 3.12. Radial club hand in Klippel–Feil syndrome.

Associated malformations are common in the Klippel–Feil syndrome. They can be visceral or skeletal. Renal abnormalities occur in one-third of patients. Congenital heart lesions, enteric cysts, and reduplication of the cord have been described.

The associated skeletal malformations are of orthopaedic interest.

Sprengel's shoulder is present in nearly one-quarter of patients with severe type I lesions. The scapula is small, elevated and may be connected to the cervical spine by a bony onovertebral bar.

Webbing of the neck may be an innocent blemish which accompanies the synostosis or may be part of Turner's syndrome coexisting with the Klippel–Feil syndrome (Turner's syndrome is gonadal hypoplasia, cubitus valgus and webbing of the neck).

Hemivertebrae and spina bifida are very common companion anomalies.

Scoliosis below the deformed neck is very common. It was seen in more than half of Hensinger's patients (Hensinger, Lang and McEwan, 1974). It is usually of the congenital variety and associated with a hemivertebra, but a progressive secondary curve can develop in an apparently normal thoracic spine. Every child with Klippel–Feil syndrome should have radiographs of the whole spine and an intravenous pyelogram. Great care must be excercised in the management of these secondary curves. Distraction methods may precipitate a neurological defect from occult neural anomalies of the cervical spine or cranial outlet such as inencephaly (Sherk, Shut and Chung, 1974).

Management of the *clinical problems* caused by the Klippel–Feil syndrome is challenging. Attempts have been made to improve appearances by bilateral upper thoracoplasty (Bonola, 1956). A Sprengel's shoulder can exaggerate shortness of the neck. The scapula can be released by extensive soft tissue release but the improvement in appearance hardly justifies the extensive dissection. No operation, however effective cosmetically, can increase movement of the cervical spine.

Problems can arise at the junctional levels between fixed and mobile segments of the spine from the degenerative disc changes produced by excessive movement. Both myelopathy and root lesions are seen (Lee and Weiss, 1981). It must be remembered that there may be associated neurological anomalies. The bony changes seen on X-ray may not be solely responsible for a deteriorating neurological picture.

Instability at the junctional segment is a greater problem than the compression of spondylosis. These patients are at risk from minor injury. Prophylactic fusion will reduce or abolish what little movement there is in the neck, but this stiffness is preferable to the tetraplegia that can follow trivial injury (Elster, 1984).

Richard III and the Klippel–Feil Syndrome
(Figure 3.13)

'I, that am curtailed of this fair proportion,
Cheated of feature by dissembling Nature,
Deformed, unfinished, sent before my time.

So lamely and unfashionable
That dogs bark at me as I halt by them.'

Shakespeare has marked England's last English king forever as a hunchbacked monster. The only authenticated contemporary portrait in the National Portrait Gallery

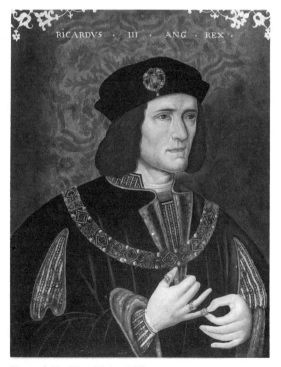

Figure 3.13. King Richard III.

shows a short neck, unfashionably long hair, the right shoulder higher than the left and a possibly hypoplastic right thumb. Shakespeare was a Tudor propagandist and as little concerned with historical truth as Winston Smith. In the late nineteenth century a wave of reaction resurrected Richard as a physically perfect hero. Lindsay's biography ascribes the portrait to Rous, whom he calls 'an unblushing timeserver' (Lindsay, 1969). Leaving aside the merits or faults of Richard as a monarch, there is conflicting evidence of his physique.

In the National Portrait Gallery are other portraits of Richard, all of which show him as deformed. Their contemporary status is doubtful and in some there is radiographic evidence to suggest that the high shoulder has been added to the original painting.

There are some contemporary written descriptions, again conflicting, and these are quoted in Markham's definitive biography.

p. 40   (Richard as a child)
'Short in stature with a delicate frame, the right shoulder being higher than the left.'

p. 124   'Not so much as to be noticeable or to cause weakness.'

p. 185   i   (quoting Rous)
'With hair down to his shoulders. Humpbacked, that his right shoulder higher than left.'

ii   (quoting Morton, *the* Morton of Morton's Fork, an unreliable witness if ever there was one)
'Left shoulder higher than right. One of his arms was withered.'

Lindsay, a less objective biographer, accepts that his right arm was disproportionately bigger, but only because he assiduously practised his sword play to match his glorious brother Edward. Professional tennis players show the same hypertrophy, and there was never any doubt as to Richard's prowess as a swordsman on the battlefield. We shall never know the truth about his physical appearance, any more than we shall ever know for certain whether he killed the Princes in the Tower. The association of an evil character with a physical deformity is an ancient misapprehension of society. What is striking is the sadness of his expression. By all accounts he was not a happy man.

Agenesis of the cervical spine

Hemivertebrae occur in the cervical spine, above, or associated with other anomalies. True agenesis of five cervical vertebrae has been reported (Nisan, Hiz and Saner, 1988). It will be remembered that Klippel and Feil described their first case as being 'par absence des vertebrae cervicales'.

Congenital spinal stenosis

Congenital narrowing of the whole cervical canal has been described. It is an entirely male phenomenon (Kessler, 1975).

Spondylolysis and spondylolisthesis

Failures of fusion between neural arch can occur on one or both sides. The pedicle can be absent (Hadley, 1946). When the defects are bilateral, forward displacement of the body can jeopardize the cord (Durbin, 1956; Guillane *et al.*, 1976).

References

Acheson, E.D. (1986) Atlanto-axial instability in people with Down's syndrome. *DHSS, SMO* 86/9.

Ahlback, S. and Collert, S. (1970) Destruction of the odontoid process due to pyogenic osteomyelitis. *Acta Radiologica*, **10**, 394.

American Academy Pediatric Committee on Sports Medicine (1984) Atlanto-axial instability in Down's syndrome. *Pediatrics*, **74**, 152.

Arnold, J. (1903) Myelocystele transposition von gewebskeimen und sympodie. *Beiträge zur Pathologischen Anatomie und zur Allgemeinen Pathologie*, **16**, 1.

Bharucha, E.P. and Dastur, H.M. (1964) Cranio-vertebral anomalies. *Brain*, **87**, 469.

Blockley, N.J. and Purser, D.W. (1956) Fractures of the odontoid process of the axis. *Journal of Bone and Joint Surgery*, **38B**, 794.

Bonola, A. (1956) Surgical treatment of the Klippel-Feil syndrome. *Journal of Bone and Joint Surgery*, **38B**, 440–449.

Burke, S.W., French, H.G. and Roberts, J.M. (1985) Chronic atlanto-axial instability in Down's syndrome. *Journal of Bone and Joint Surgery*, **67A**, 1356.

Chiari, H. (1891) Ueber verändervungen des kleinhirns in folge von hydrocephalie des grosshirns. *Deutsche Medizinische Wochenschrift*, **17**, 1172.

Crockard, A. and Ransford, A. (1985) One stage transoral decompression and posterior stabilization in cervical myelopathy. *Journal of Bone and Joint Surgery*, **67B**, 498.

Davidson, R.G. (1988) Atlanto-axial instability in Down's syndrome. *Pediatrics*, **81**, 857.

Durbin, F. (1956) Spondylolisthesis of the cervical spine. *Journal of Bone and Joint Surgery*, **38B**, 734.

Elster, A.D. (1984) Quadriplegia after minor trauma in the Klippel Feil syndrome. *Journal of Bone and Joint Surgery*, **66A**, 1473.

Feil, A.L. (1919) L'absence et la diminution des vertibres cervicales. *Theses de Paris.*

Fielding, J.W. (1965) Disappearance of the central portion of the odontoid process. *Journal of Bone and Joint Surgery*, **47A**, 1228.

Fielding, J.W. and Griffin, P.P. (1974) Os odontoideum. *Journal of Bone and Joint Surgery*, **56A**, 187.

Fielding, J.W., Hensinger, R.N. and Hawkins, R.J. (1980) Os odontoideum. *Journal of Bone and Joint Surgery*, **62A**, 376.

Finerman, G.A., Sakai, D. and Weingarten, S. (1976) Atlanto-axial dislocation in a mongoloid child. *Journal of Bone and Joint Surgery*, **58A**, 408.

Freiberger, R.H., Wilson, P.D. and Nicholas, J.A. (1965) Acquired absence of the odontoid process. *Journal of Bone and Joint Surgery*, **47A**, 1231.

Garber, J.N. (1964) Abnormalities of the atlas and axis. *Journal of Bone and Joint Surgery*, **46A**, 1782.

Geehr, R.N., Rothman, S.L.G. and Kier, E.L. (1978) The role of CT in the evaluation of upper cervical spine pathology. *Computed tomography*, **2**, 79.

Gillman, C.L. (1959) Congenital absence of the odontoid process. *Journal of Bone and Joint Surgery*, **41A**, 340.

Guillane, J., Roulleau, J., Fardou, H., Trail, J. and Manelfe, C. (1976) Congenital spondylolysis of cervical vertebrae with spondylolisthesis. *Neuroradiology*, **11**, 159.

Gunderson, C.H., Greenspan, R.H., Glaser, G.H. and Lubs, H.A. (1967) The Klippel Feil syndrome. *Medicine*, **46**, 491.

Gwinn, J.L. and Smith, J.L. (1962) Acquired and congenital absence of the odontoid process. *American Journal of Roentgenology*, **88**, 424.

Hadley, L.A. (1946) Congenital absence of pedicle from cervical vertebrae. *American Journal of Roentgenology*, **55**, 193.

Hamblen, D. (1967) Occipito-cervical fusion. *Journal of Bone and Joint Surgery*, **49B**, 33.

Hensinger, R.N., Lang, J.E. and MacEwan, D. (1974) The Klippel Feil syndrome. *Journal of Bone and Joint Surgery*, **56A**, 1246.

Jeffreys, T.E. (1980) *Disorders of the Cervical Spine* Butterworths. London, p. 37.

Kessler, J.T. (1975) Congenital narrowing of the cervical spinal canal. *Journal of Neurology, Neurosurgery and Psychiatry*, **38**, 1218.

Klein, R.A., Snyder, R.A. and Schwartz, J.H. (1976) Lateral medullary syndrome in a child. *Journal of the American Medical Association*, **253**, 940.

Klippel, M. and Feil, A.L. (1912) Anomalie de la colonne vertebrale par absence des vertebrae cervicales. *Bulletin Société Anthropologie, Paris*, **65**, 101.

Lee, C.K. and Weiss, A.B. (1981) Isolated congenital cervical block vertebrae below the axis with neurological symptoms. *Spine*, **6**, 118.

Lindsay, P. (1969) *King Richard III.* Howard Baker

Lloyd Roberts, G.C. (1971) *Orthopaedics in Infancy and Childhood.* **44**, 136. Butterworths, London.

McKeever, F.M. (1968) Atlanto-axial instability. *Surgery Clinics of North America*, **48**, 1375.

McRae, D.L. (1953) Bony abnormalities in the region of the foramen magnum. *Acta Radiologica*, **40**, 335.

Markham, C.R. (1973) *Richard III. His Life and Character.* Cedric Chivers. pp. 40, 124, 185.

Michaels, L., Prevost, M.J. and Croug, D.F. (1989) Pathological changes in a case of os odontoideum. *Journal of Bone and Joint Surgery*, **51A**, 965.

Michie, I. and Clark, M. (1968) Neurological syndromes associated with cervical and cranio-cervical anomalies. *Archives of Neurology*, **18**, 241.

Minderhoud, J.M., Brakman, R. and Penning, L. (1969) Os odontoideum. *Journal of Neurological Sciences*, **8**, 521.

Nicholson, J.S. and Sherk, H.H. (1968) Abnormalities of the occipito-cervical junction. *Journal of Bone and Joint Surgery*, **50A**, 295.

Nisan, N., Hiz, M. and Saner, H. (1988) Total agenesis of five cervical vertebrae. *Journal of Bone and Joint Surgery*, **70B**, 668.

Okada, K., Kagawa, T.F., Yonenobo, K. and Ono, K. (1980) Cervical diastametomyelia with a stable neurological defect. *Journal of Bone and Joint Surgery*, **68A**, 934.

Prosick, V.R., Samberg, L.C. and Wesolowski, D.P. (1985) Klippel-Feil syndrome associated with spinal stenosis. *Journal of Bone and Joint Surgery*, **67A**, 6.

Schiff, D.C.M. and Parke, W.W. (1972) Arterial blood supply of the odontoid process. *Anatomical Record*, **172**, 399.

Seimon, L. (1977) Fracture of the odontoid process in young children. *Journal of Bone and Joint Surgery*, **59A**, 943.

Shepard, C.N. (1966) Familial hypoplasia of the odontoid process. *Journal of Bone and Joint Surgery*, **48A**, 1224.

Sherk, H.H. and Nicholson, J.T. (1969) Rotatory atlanto-axial dislocation with ossiculum terminale and mongolism. *Journal of Bone and Joint Surgery*, **51A**, 957.

Sherk, H.H., Shut, L. and Chung, S. (1974) Inencephalic deformity of the cervical spine with Klippel-Feil anomalies and congenital elevation of the scapula. *Journal of Bone and Joint Surgery*, **56A**, 1254–1259.

Sinto, G. and Pandya, S.K. (1968) Treatment of congenital atlanto-axial dislocation. *Proceedings of the Australian Association of Neurology*, **5**, 507.

Spillane, J.D., Pallis, C. and Jones, A.M. (1957) Developmental anomalies in the region of the foramen magnum. *Brain*, **80**, 11.

Taylor, A.R. and Byrnes, D.P. (1974) Foramen magnum and high cervical cord compression. *Brain*, **97**, 473.

Torklus, von D. and Gehle, W. (1972) *The Upper Cervical Spine*. Butterworths, London, p. 45.

Tredwell, S.S. and O'Brien, J.P. (1975) Avascular necrosis of the proximal end of the dens. *Journal of Bone and Joint Surgery*, **57A**, 332.

Wallenberg, A. (1897) Embolie der arterie cerebellaris postero-inferior sinistra. *Archivs fur Psychologie*, **27**, 204.

Wynne-Davies, R., Hall, C.M., Howell, C.J. *et al.* (1989) Instability of the upper cervical spine. *Skeletal Dysplasia Group for Teaching and Research*. Unpublished.

4 Fractures and dislocations of the neck

Robert G. Pringle

'For he fell from the seat and his neck brake, and he
died, for he was an old man, and heavy.'

1 Samuel IV 17.

Introduction

In this chapter the common injuries of the
cervical spinal skeleton are discussed and
the more unusual varieties considered
briefly. Of paramount importance in their
assessment and management is the presence
or absence of associated spinal cord injury,
as any injury to the cord, however slight,
renders it significantly more vulnerable to
hypotension and hypoxia. Where there is no
cord injury, management may be conservative or operative, according to the wishes of
the patient and the experience of the
surgeon, whereas in the presence of cord
injury, protection of the cord and management of the associated neural deficit must
take precedence.

The number of spinal cord injuries has
increased world-wide in the last 30 years
(Gehrig and Michaelis, 1968; Michaelis, 1976)
particularly in the more developed countries
where road traffic accidents are the major
cause. At present the incidence in the UK is
estimated at 10–15 patients per million population per annum. This, together with improved
resuscitation and general medical and nursing
care in specialist centres has led to an ever
increasing number of severely disabled
survivors of middle and high cervical injuries.
The financial implications are considerable
and while the care of the patient is the
surgeon's primary concern, the rise in cost to
the Health Service imposes a further responsi-
bility upon him or her (Young, 1978).

The severity of neural injury is often
unrelated to that of the spinal column, and
tetraplegia may occur in the absence of
evident bone or joint damage, most commonly
in children and the elderly. These catastrophic
injuries which leave the mind so clear and the
patient entirely dependent on others raise
great moral and social problems. The ethical
aspects have been considered by Walsh (1967).

Epidemiology

While road traffic accidents remain the major
cause of spinal injury in most countries, with
falls the second, this is not always the case, and
the varying incidence and aetiology around the
world provide an interesting reflection of social
behaviour. Thus in Greenland the most
common cause is attempted suicide (Pederson,
Muller and Biering-Sorensen, 1989), while in
South India falls from trees account for 55 per
cent, falling weights 18.4 per cent and road
accidents 12.8 per cent (Chacko et al., 1986). In
the Beijing area of China, road accidents
account for less than 10 per cent, compared with
falls (30 per cent) (Wang et al., 1990). In Zaria,
Nigeria, 'collapsing mud walls' come second to
road accidents (Iwegbu, 1983). In the USA gun
and stab wounds are the third most common
cause (15 per cent) (Collins, 1983). The position
is similar in Brazil, where, however, diving
accidents are equal third (Masini, Neto and
Neves, 1990). However, in Chicago stab wounds
are the second most common cause (22 per

cent) of spinal cord injury in general, and the most common cause (16 per cent) of paraplegia (Yarkony *et al.*, 1990).

Dealing specifically with cervical injuries, (Ersmark, Dalen and Kalen, 1990) reported from Sweden an incidence of 50 per cent road accident victims and 37 per cent falls, while Stover and Fine (USA 1987) reported that of the spinal cord injuries in their series 50 per cent occurred on the roads, 20 per cent in falls, 15 per cent acts of violence, 15 per cent sport, and of that total 52 per cent were cervical and 48 per cent dorsal and lumbar injuries. Of the cervical injuries approximately half were complete.

Industrial injury, at least in the UK, is exceeded now as a cause by domestic accidents to older people. At the other end of life neonatal injuries following delivery form a very small but interesting group (Allen, 1976).

Sports injuries have become an increasing problem as ever more people of all ages undertake increasingly dangerous leisure activities. Rugby football is a notable cause of cervical tragedy, and we admit on average one rugby player a year with important cervical cord injury, often tetraplegia. Silver (1987) reported 68 rugby injuries in 7700 patients compared with 16 trampoline and 38 gymnastic injuries, while Williams and McKibbin (1979) described nine serious neck injuries in four playing seasons. Four of these players remained paralysed.

Diving in shallow pools and rivers in the UK and on holiday abroad is a more potent cause of major cervical injury to the British population than is rugby (Figure 4.1), while horse riding and motor cycle sports also contribute to the total. Not surprisingly, skiing in Switzerland, football in the USA (Schneider *et al.*, 1961, 1970; Schneider, 1966; Funk and Wells, 1975) and wrestling in Turkey (Acikgoz, Ozgen and Erbengi, 1990) take their respective toll on the spinal cord.

Iatrogenic causes, for example following chiropractic manipulation (Pratt-Thomas and Berger, 1947; Livingston, 1971), and inadequate initial care (Sussman, 1978) with their associated medico-legal implications should be noted.

Prevention

General measures aimed at reducing the road toll including the control of speed limits and

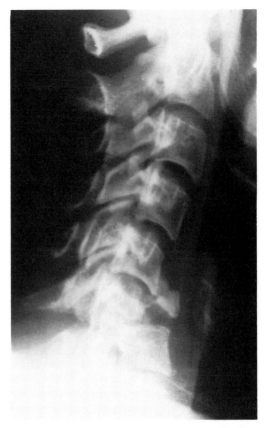

Figure 4.1. Burst fracture C6. A typical diving injury. Complete tetraplegia.

alcohol abuse must contribute to a reduction in the number of serious neck injuries (McDermott, 1978) and head restraints help to minimize the effect of rear end collisions, but the role of the seat belt in relationship to neck injury is less clear. Watson (1983) confidently reported a reduction in the expected frequency of injury to seat-belted occupants, but was reporting on spinal cord injuries in general admitted to a Spinal Injury Unit.

Ackroyd and Hobbs (1979) reported a substantial decrease in major injuries with the use of seat belts, but that minor neck injuries were increased. This would agree with our own experience. Both flexion rotation and compression injuries are commonly seen in seat-belted occupants of vehicles involved in frontal collisions or which have overturned. Many such victims have cervical root lesions only but major cord injury may still result.

Much attention has been given to the reframing of the laws of rugby, stricter refereeing, neck strenthening exercises, and the avoidance of physical mismatches in an attempt to reduce the incidence of neck injury (Yeo, 1983 personal communication; Silver, 1986 personal communication), but with limited success. Tragedies continue to occur. More could be done to increase public awareness of the dangers of diving into shallow water and of 'drinking and diving'. Early moves towards a publicity campaign along these lines have been made recently in the UK (Frankel, 1989 personal communication).

First aid

Awareness and appropriate first aid on the rugby field and elsewhere would minimize cord injury and reduce the level of permanent disability (Piggot, 1989 personal communication).

Moving the patient from the scene of the accident to hospital requires special care to prevent any movement which might increase the displacement and further endanger the cord. At least four people, preferably five, are needed to lift the patient 'in one piece' in the supine position onto a firm stretcher. The most experienced attendant should apply continuous gentle traction to the head and neck and take command of the whole operation. The head and neck should be kept in a straight line with the long axis of the body, and great care should be taken to prevent twisting or bending the neck. All activities are carried out in unison and with the greatest gentleness. With an unconscious patient in respiratory distress the lateral or semi-lateral position is acceptable provided an improvised roll or pack is placed between the shoulder and the neck.

In certain circumstances transport by air to a specialized centre is life saving, a point made by Wannamaker (1954) in the context of the Korean war. Gregg (1967) and Hachen (1974) advocate the use of medical teams and helicopter services for certain geographical situations. Neurological deterioration during transportation and after admission to hospital has been reported (Rogers, 1957; Geisler, Wynne Jones and Jousse, 1966). Toscano (1988) in a large Australian study found evidence of such deterioration between the

time of the accident and arrival in the Spinal Injuries Unit in 25 per cent of cases. While much of this deterioration may be attributed to the inevitable progression of the pathological process, some undoubtedly is due to inadequate primary care.

Mechanisms of injury

1 Spinal column injury

Injuries to the cervical spine are usually caused by indirect violence transmitted through the head and producing movements which transgress the normal range. Alternatively, forces applied to the trunk may cause excessive neck movement by sudden acceleration or deceleration of the head. Direct injuries are caused by blows on the neck resulting in fractures of the neural arch. Missile injuries are included in this category.

It is customary to recognize five major forces. These are flexion, extension, rotation, compression and shear forces. Unfortunately these terms are liable to misinterpretation. Roaf (1972) points out that extension or hyperextension really means an increase in length – that is the opposite of compression. Braakman and Penning (1976) prefer the term 'hyperanteflexion' for flexion to distinguish it from 'hyperdeflexion' or extension. Convention rather than scientific accuracy has sanctioned the terms used in this chapter.

Ideally each deforming force should be classified according to its principal direction, its subsidiary direction, and should take into account distraction compression and rotation. On this basis Roaf has suggested a comprehensive classification using the principles of elementary dynamics and conventional mathematical notations.

One of the difficulties in any classification of spinal injuries is that external forces are modified by intrinsic factors such as the varying strength of the bones and ligaments at different ages and whether the protective muscles are 'on guard' or relaxed at the time of injury. While it is often possible to deduce the mechanism of injury from a study of the X-rays, the different deforming forces may produce similar pictures and secondary displacements may confuse the issue. Nevertheless, with the physical findings (location of bruise marks, scalp wounds, facial injuries) the radiographs and the history of the accident in mind it is usually possible to build up a mental picture of how the injury was caused. The objective is to distinguish between injuries in which flexion is the predominant force and those caused by hyperextension. If an extension injury is mistaken for a flexion injury and the neck is treated in hyperextension dire consequences may result. At the same time it should be recognized that the vertebral injury is rarely the result of a single force and that compression and rotation are important components of many injuries.

In the attempt to reach a better understanding of these problems one of the earlier experimenters (Schmaus, 1890) produced concussion in the spinal cord of the rabbit by delivering repeated blows to a board securely attached to the animal's back. Since then other workers have used both animal and human cadaveric spines under various stresses and compression forces. Roaf (1960) could not produce a rupture of normal spinal ligaments by hyperextension or hyperflexion, but when rotation or horizontal shearing forces were added ligamentous rupture and dislocation readily occurred.

Selecki and Williams (1970) carried out an extensive study on 22 cadaveric cervical spines using complete blocks from the first thoracic vertebra to the base of the skull. A hydraulic jack was used to exert pressure on the specimen which was clamped between metal plates. They found that the major injuries were accompanied by direct or indirect evidence of severe damage to the vertebral, radicular or anterior spinal arteries. In specimens subjected to hyperextension, the site of injury was most commonly in the lower cervical spine. In particular circumstances, hyperextension forces produced fracture dislocations in the upper cervical spine. Flexion forces caused injuries above C5. They advised that skull traction should be used as the initial measure in all fracture dislocations, irrespective of the mechanism of injury. Skull traction should not be employed in hyperextension injuries with no fracture or dislocation. This excellent monograph should be consulted for the detailed clinical findings.

Using a similar apparatus with lateral cineradiography Bauze and Ardran (1978) made a number of observations. They showed that when the lower part of the spine was fixed and slightly flexed and the upper cervical spine extended and free to move, a vertical compression force would then produce bilateral facetal dislocation in the lower cervical spine without fracture. They referred to an earlier study in which Cornish (1968) describes the 'ducking' position of the neck in a person anticipating a blow on the top of the head. The attitude is one of mid and lower cervical flexion with capital extension. Forward dislocation resulted from a combination of vertical compression, and flexion and horizontal shearing forces at the junction of the fixed and mobile parts of the spine.

Beatson (1963) showed that unilateral facetal dislocation (locked facet) could only occur if the corresponding interspinous ligament and the capsule of the posterior facet joint was completely torn. (We have confirmed this on more than one occasion at surgery.) He found as a rule that there was only minor damage to the annulus. In producing bilateral facet locking it was necessary to rupture the capsules of both facet joints, the interspinous ligament, and the posterior longitudinal ligament. At the same time he carried out an interesting radiographic study using wire markers inserted into the facets of adjacent vertebrae. On the true lateral X-ray forward dislocation of a vertebral body on the one below by more than half the anteroposterior width of the body, suggests dislocation of both facet joints (Figure 4.2). A forward slip of less than half the anteroposterior depth indicates a unilateral facet dislocation (Figure 4.3). We have found this a satisfactory working rule, although obviously further X-rays including oblique views should be taken.

2 Spinal cord and nerve root injury

Even with gross vertebral displacement the spinal cord and nerve roots may escape injury (Pitman, Pitman and Greenberg, 1977). Conversely, functionally complete cord lesions may occur in the absence of recognizable bony or ligamentous damage. In some elderly spondylotic patients and in children, serious neurological damage may occur with normal radiological appearances. We have examined many of our younger tetraplegic patients years after injury without finding evidence of skeletal

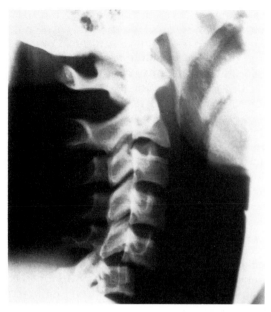

Figure 4.2. Bilateral facet dislocation. Displacement more than half body width.

damage. Similar remarks apply to the tetraparesis often encountered in block vertebrae and other congenital anomalies. Certain types of injury, however, are known to be commonly associated with recognizable patterns of neurological damage (Cheshire, 1969).

Bilateral facet dislocation is commonly accompanied by a complete cord lesion, while in unilateral facet dislocation nerve root injury alone is more common. Severe compression injuries, notably burst fractures of a vertebral body (Holdsworth, 1970), and at least one type of 'tear drop' fracture (Schneider, 1955) usually result in anterior cord syndrome.

The exceptions from this rule form an interesting and at times puzzling group. We have seen many patients with complete bilateral dislocation, not uncommonly missed for several weeks, whose only complaint has been stiffness and discomfort in the neck, or minor sensory symptoms in one or both upper limbs (Figure 4.4). The correlation between the

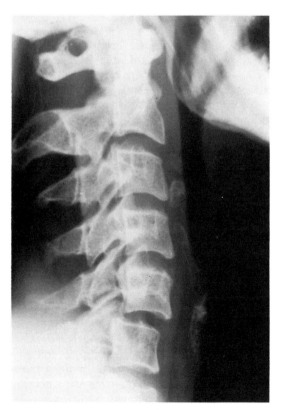

Figure 4.3. Unilateral facet dislocation. Displacement less than half body width.

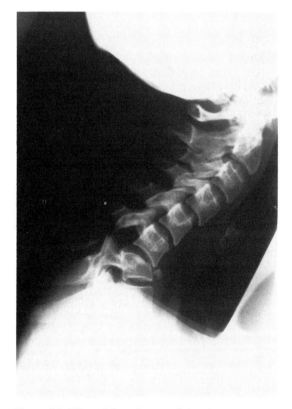

Figure 4.4. Bilateral facet fracture dislocation undiagnosed for four weeks. No cord injury.

vertebral displacement and the neural damage remains elusive, but certain factors must be mentioned.

In some fracture dislocations posterior element fracture may lead to detachment of the neural arch – in effect a traumatic spondylolysis – resulting in 'instantaneous laminectomy' thus protecting the cord from being crushed between the margin of the lamina and the posterior aspect of the body of the adjacent vertebra (Figure 4.5). Breig (1978) has shown that the cervical cord shortens in extension, and reduction in tension in this fashion may explain some of these unusual cases of cord sparing also.

The increased vulnerability of the cord and nerve roots in spinal stenosis has long been recognized. We are all familiar with the astonishing variations in the facial and body features of the human race, and it would be surprising if these were not mirrored in the dimensions of the spinal canal, epidural space, and spinal cord. Elliott (1945) noted the wide variations in spinal cord diameter. The transverse diameter of the spinal canal below the third cervical vertebra is larger than the sagittal, and it is variation in the latter that is crucial to the integrity of the cord. The normal average diameter of the mid-cervical spine has been shown to be approximately 17 mm, and Arnold (1955) reported the range at C6 to be between 13 and 22 mm. A sagittal diameter of 13–15 mm is considered diagnostic of stenosis and has been found to be associated with transient tetraparesis following soft tissue injury in young athletes (Ladd and Scranton, 1986, Torg *et al.*, 1986).

In a majority of patients the cord and nerve root damage occurs at the time of injury, that is to say in practical terms the neural damage is coincident with the injury and its clinical manifestations are maximal at that time. This does not preclude the well recognized phenomenon of ascent (usually temporary) of one or two segments, presumably due to increasing oedema, or the worsening of the neural deficit by inept management. The cord may be injured by bony displacement which reduces the sagittal diameter of the canal or by the retropulsion of bone fragments from a vertebral body shattered by a severe compression injury. Whatever the exact mechanism, it is the severity of the initial injury which dictates the neurological outcome, the latter being, in general, independent of the X-ray appearances, the method of management (provided it is competent), and even the restoration of normal skeletal anatomy (Dall, 1972).

Animal studies have demonstrated that the pathological changes are related to the severity of the trauma. The first histological changes occur in the grey matter within 5 minutes of injury. Small haemorrhages appear within 1 hour, and central ischaemic and haemorrhagic lesions are clearly present within 4 hours, followed by progressive grey matter necrosis (Figure 4.6).

Changes in the white matter commence 3–4 hours after injury, initially as oedema and with disordered perfusion, leading to destruction of the white matter within a matter of days. In more severe lesions, however, diffuse haemorrhages may be seen throughout both grey and white matter within 2 hours of injury. This has been noted in post-mortem studies. Oedema begins within 5 minutes, is maximal at 5 days, and regresses over 15 days or more. The fluid

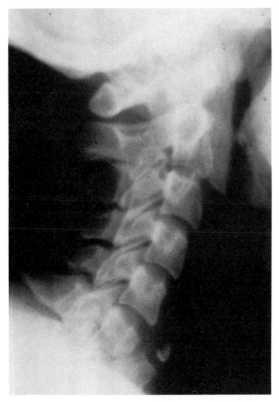

Figure 4.5. Traumatic spondylolisthesis C7. No neurology. Uneventful healing in situ with conservative treatment.

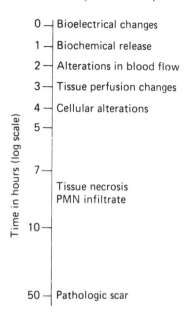

0 ─┤ Bioelectrical changes
1 ─┤ Biochemical release
2 ─┤ Alterations in blood flow
3 ─┤ Tissue perfusion changes
4 ─┤ Cellular alterations
5 ─┤

7 ─┤

    Tissue necrosis
    PMN infiltrate

10 ─┤

50 ─┤ Pathologic scar

Time in hours (log scale)

Figure 4.6. Pathophysiological changes that take place as the result of a spinal cord injury. From Ducker (1976).

may originate from ruptured vessels, disrupted cells, CSF originally in the subarachnoid space and altered vascular permeability (Ducker, 1976; Jellinger, 1976).

Immediately following injury there is a loss of vasomotor response of the injuried segment, and a rising PCO_2 no longer leads to vasodilation, leading in turn to relative ischaemia and hypoxia. Studies in spinal cord perfusion have led to the suggestion that injury stimulates the release of a toxic substance in the cord which may contribute to the destructive process.

Once the area of central haemorrhagic necrosis is established it is self perpetuating. Depending on the severity of injury it may spread rostrally and caudally over a few segments, or in exceptional cases involve the greater part of the spinal cord. Although the pathological changes are progressive over the first week, clinical improvement in the neurological state nonetheless may commence in that time. The complexity of the subject and the many pitfalls of experimental studies have been pointed out by Yeo, Payne and Hinwood (1975) and Yeo (1976) in their comprehensive work on sheep. However, no experimental studies have produced convincing evidence, or evidence reproducible in clinical practice, that any physical or chemical manipulation of the cord can enhance the rate or degree of neurological recovery. Certainly, treatment with steroids or antiadrenergic blocking agents, spinal cord cooling and perfusion, and surgery such as myelotomy have all been tried and found wanting. Hyperbaric oxygen has been found to be of some value in animal work, but has yet to be established in clinical practice (Yeo, Stabback and Mackenzie, 1977).

From the pathological studies one would conclude that if medical or surgical manipulation of the condition is to modify its course, such manipulation must be carried out within the first few hours of injury. Humans can withstand moderate degrees of grey matter destruction in the cord, but if there is a period of time immediately following injury when the white matter could be salvaged, this might alter the whole course of cord injury. In 1990, Bracken *et al.* published the results of a multi-centre trial which indicated that methylprednisolone given within 8 hours of injury improves neurological recovery. This study did not show whether the improved neurological recovery was of functional significance. Independent confirmation of the results is awaited.

Injury to the vertebral artery has been described at post mortem by Vanezis (1989) in 31 per cent of 32 road accident victims suspected of having some form of posterior neck trauma. The highest incidence was in the upper cervical spine, and incomplete tears were most common, sometimes with subarachnoid haemorrhage. More recently, Louw *et al.* (1990) reported vertebral artery occlusion (one bilateral) in nine of 12 consecutive cases of unilateral and bilateral facet dislocations after reduction. The level of occlusion was that of the dislocated facet in only three cases, and two (both at C5/6) had neurological deficit cranial to the level of injury. At present this information has no therapeutic implications, but may provide some explanation of the not uncommon finding of associated cranial nerve lesions in high spinal injury (Grundy, McSweeney and Francis Jones, 1984).

The role of the intervertebral disc in acute injuries is still disputed. Jefferson (1940) believed that the disc was a common compressive agent, and Taylor and Blackwood (1948) believed that myelography should demonstrate this. In the event this did not prove to be the case. More recently MRI scanning has proved valuable in delineating disc pathology in spinal cord injury, although whether this will contribute significantly to the management remains to be seen. In general there is no convincing evidence that disc protrusion plays an important part in the condition or that removal of the disc can modify its progress. Apple, McDonald and Smith (1987) in a retrospective study, found only five cases of symptomatic herniated disc in 657 cervical cord injuries. Of these, three had bilateral facet dislocations, and four incomplete syndromes and radicular pain. However Cloward (1961), Norrell (1971), Pierce (1969) and Pierce and Nickel (1977) differ. Our own experience is similar to that of Apple *et al.*

Ransohoff (1977) attempted to put the whole problem into perspective by saying, 'if, however, external compression of the cervical spinal cord can be clearly documented, it would seem to represent a violation of surgical principles not to recommend removal of this offending mass at the earliest possible moment if the patient's general condition is sufficiently stable to undergo surgical intervention'. If the spinal canal has been realigned by skull traction or reposition, this statement perhaps overlooks the probability that it was the forces of injury, already spent, which initiated the subsequent self-destructive process in the neural tissue.

Nerve root injury may follow compression in the intervertebral foramen, or result from the indirect injury of traction. According to Hadley (1944, 1949), the roots occupy about one-quarter of the intervertebral canal and are cushioned by loose connective tissue in the dural sleeve. We have been surprised by the quality of root recovery even when the dislocation remains unreduced. Primary associated brachial plexus injuries and root avulsions imply a poor prognosis (Bonney, 1959) and many months may elapse before the limits of such a lesion and the prognosis can be defined (Schaafsma, 1970). Sunderland (1974) offers a masterly review of this complex problem.

Process of repair

Vertebral column

Injuries to the vertebral bodies heal rapidly by endosteal and subperiosteal bone formation. Fractures of the transverse processes and spinous processes are slow to unite and often fail to heal. Where there is much bony damage, eventual stability is almost certain, in contrast to predominantly ligamentous disruptions where persistent instability is often a feature.

The terms stability and instability are confusing when applied to a structure which is inherently mobile – secure or unsafe might be more appropriate words. Cheshire's (1969) definition is useful. He defined stability as 'the absence of any abnormal mobility between any pair of vertebrae, with or without pain or other clinical manifestations, when lateral X-rays of the cervical spine are taken in flexion and extension at the conclusion of the conservative treatment of a fracture or a fracture dislocation'.

It is safest to regard all cervical injuries as unstable in the early days, until clinical assessment and radiological examination establishes the true state of affairs. The term 'instability' clearly is a relative one and should not be equated with the necessity to fuse the cervical spine. Injuries which are initially unstable may in a reasonable time stabilize. While experience shows that certain injuries are inherently unstable, there are no absolute rules for predicting ultimate stability. Much depends on the forces of injury, the neurological status, the method of treatment, the time of immobilization, and the patient's mobility and general healing power.

White, Southwick and Panjabi (1976) have added greatly to our knowledge of instability 'and clarification of this subject'. They quote a final instability rate of about 10 per cent following dislocations of the lower cervical spine. Unfortunately these figures, taken from a large series, did not differentiate between the various anatomical lesions.

Cheshire (1969) found a late instability rate of between 4.8 and 7.3 per cent in the main groups, in contrast to anterior subluxation where the late instability rate was 21 per cent. In a small series (McSweeney, 1971), where the cord injury was incomplete, there were only two cases of late instability. Twenty-five patients had suffered unilateral dislocations, 18 bilateral and seven were compression injuries. Paradoxically, the two unstable injuries were in this last group.

Spinal cord

The gross changes depend on the severity of injury and the time lapse. The early infarction of the grey matter is gradually replaced by a dense felting of neuroglia. This reaction is well established in the early weeks after injury and is usually more extensive longitudinally. In severe injuries the scar tissue becomes increasingly impenetrable and degenerative cyst formation is common at and remote from the site of injury. Regeneration of some fibres is well documented (Windle, 1955) and the long held belief that axonal regeneration does not occur has been disproved on many occasions. Wolman (1964) reviewed the subject and indicated the direction of future research. However, at present and for the foreseeable future, the very limited regenerative powers of the spinal cord are not clinically useful, and reconstruction and repair remain experimental procedures only.

Clinical features

'The facility with which severe cervical cord trauma may be sustained is only surpassed by the ease with which such damage can be overlooked.' (J.B. Cook.)

A complaint of pain in the neck following an accident should arouse suspicion of a cervical injury. This is especially so if the accident was of a nature known to be associated with spinal damage, and accompanied at the time by electric-shock-like feelings in the limbs. Unconscious patients, those who have fallen from a height, and the victims of traffic accidents are always suspect.

The patient may walk into the Accident Department supporting the head with their hands, or the only complaint may be of some minor discomfort and stiffness in the neck. Pain in the scalp over the occipital region may be a presenting symptom in upper cervical injuries. Pain, weakness or alteration in sensation in the upper limb or head should alert the examiner to the possibility of a unilateral facet dislocation. Patients who have sustained an incomplete cord injury may complain of stiffness rather than inability to move the lower limbs. Special care should be exercised with older patients who have tripped or fallen down stairs. Hyperextension injuries accompanied by a central cord syndrome are missed with monotonous regularity. Retention of urine may be a clue.

The diagnosis of tetraplegia should not present difficulties. Diaphragmatic breathing with paralysis of the intercostal muscles, the posture of the limbs, a warm dry skin and a slow full pulse, especially if accompanied by a low blood pressure, should draw attention to the neck.

A detailed history of the accident often helps in assessing the magnitude and direction of the injuring force. It is sometimes difficult to decide whether the patient moved his limbs immediately following the accident. This important point should be checked with the witnesses as well as with the victim. It is often a vital factor in prognosis.

General examination

The patient should be examined in a quiet area, lying on the back on gentle long axis traction, or with the neck immobilized between sandbags. Associated injuries should be assessed. In traffic accidents these may be life threatening and take precedence over the cervical injuries. More usually, as in recreational accidents, associated injuries are of a trivial nature. The location of bruise marks, lacerations and areas of tenderness should be carefully noted. These may give a clue to the direction of the injuring force. Swelling of the neck is usually an ominous sign, but in contrast to lumbar injuries palpation seldom reveals a gap between the vertebral processes.

Muscle spasm, tilting of the head, and alteration of the bitemporal or interpupillary line (Ravichandran, 1978) merit further investigation. The back as well as the front of the patient must always be examined. Mistakes arise most commonly because the possibility of a cervical injury is not considered.

Neurological examination

This aims to establish the presence and level of cord injury, whether the lesion is complete or incomplete, and the nature and extent of any root involvement. The primary assessment and each examination should be carefully documented. Cross checking with a colleague's independent observations is helpful. Early treatment is planned in the light of the neurological findings and even at this stage a realistic rehabilitation programme can be outlined.

It is generally unwise to discuss the prognosis in complete lesions with the patient until some weeks have elapsed, but a responsible relative should be appraised of the situation. The examination follows the time honoured procedure of assessing the state of consciousness, the extent of any sensory or voluntary motor loss, and reflex alterations. It is repeated at frequent intervals without fatiguing the patient and in the light of the initial findings.

Sensory examination

This should include the modalities of light touch, pin prick, vibration and joint position sense. Testing for alterations in thermal sensation can be deferred until later.

Proceed from the innnervated to the denervated areas, observing whether there is a band of hyperaesthesia and outlining the area with a skin pencil. This indicates the level of the cord lesion, or the territory of any involved nerve root(s) where the cord is intact. In the acute phase it is easier to determine which roots are intact, than to distinguish root damage which is often incomplete and associated with hyperaesthesia from the disturbance caused by the cord injury. The occipital area of the scalp (C2), the front of the neck (C3) and upper chest (C4) must be examined.

It is important to note that the posterior rami of C4 supply the skin below the clavicles and along this area are contiguous with the T2 dermatomes. Not a few lower cervical lesions have been referred to our Unit incorrectly diagnosed by experienced surgeons as upper dorsal on this basis (and because even complete C6 lesions may still achieve trick movements of the fingers by wrist dorsiflexion).

Sensory impairment in the upper limbs is noted over the shoulders (C5) on the outer aspect of the forearm, thumb, index and middle fingers (C6), in the ring and little fingers (C7), and along the ulnar border of the hand and forearm (C8). Preservation of sensation along the inner aspect of the arm and in the axilla indicates that the first and second thoracic segments are intact. Having established the sensory level, attention is then directed to the rest of the body and in particular to the sacral area and perineum. Appreciation of light touch and pin prick should be carefully assessed. The patient must be rolled onto the side while traction on the neck is maintained and the spine kept aligned, and later the lower limbs abducted. Preservation of sensation over the sacral area and in the perineum offers reassuring evidence that the cord injury is incomplete.

The importance of this examination taken in conjunction with the anal skin reflex and the bulbocavernosus reflex cannot be overemphasized. The latter is elicited by squeezing the glans penis or by pressure on the clitoris, while noting the contraction of the anal sphincter on the gloved finger. The anal 'wink' is evoked by a pin prick on the anal skin. Both reflexes are cord mediated and are in abeyance during the stage of spinal shock. This absence of all reflex activity below the level of the cord injury usually lasts for 24 hours or so. Reappearance of one or other of these two reflexes heralds the end of spinal shock.

If there is no sensory sparing or evidence of voluntary muscle power below the level of the cord injury, in the presence of an anal skin reflex or a positive bulbocavernosus reflex, then the cord lesion is complete. There are few exceptions to this rule. While it is reasonable to wait for 48 hours from the time of injury before reaching this conclusion, patients judged to have a complete lesion by this criterion are unlikely to make a useful functional recovery below its level. Priapism and protracted flexion of the great toe on plantar stimulation (malignant Strumpell reflex) are ominous signs.

Motor examination

In the initial examination group (joint) movement rather than individual muscle action should be tested. Apparent weakness due to pain and apprehension should be noted. The paralysis of cord injury is characterized by its myotome distribution. Muscle testing is carried out in sequence with the following key levels as a guide – deltoid and biceps (C5), extensor of the wrist (C6), triceps, pronator teres and flexor carpi radialis (C7), finger flexors (C8) and intrinsic muscles of the hand (T1). More distal sparing is then sought with special reference to the toe flexors and the anterior tibial muscle. The discovery of any voluntary muscle power below the expected level of injury is an indication that the lesion is incomplete as is sensory preservation below that level.

Examination of the reflexes

The deep tendon reflexes and the superficial abdominal and cremasteric reflexes are tested, but are seldom present at this stage. The early return of the tendon reflexes is a hopeful sign. The importance of the perineal cord mediated reflexes has been stressed. The routine is completed by examination of the cranial nerves and the autonomic system. High cervical injuries are sometimes associated with impairment of sensation on the face. Horner's syndrome, dryness of the throat, conjunctivitis, meteorism, and impaired sphincter control are indications of autonomic dysfunction.

Observations on the neurological picture

Intelligent appraisal of the neurological examination offers the best guide to the future and any evidence that the injury is incomplete alters the whole prognosis. It has been pointed out that when the patient is immediately tetraplegic, and if the signs remain those of a complete lesion during the first 48 hours, no useful functional recovery of more than one or two segments below the level of cord injury can be expected.

Incomplete lesions may result in localized damage affecting discrete parts of the cord or a more diffuse pathology, but insufficient to result in complete loss of function. Guttmann (1973) described the various syndromes, but in the early days after injury it is often difficult to classify the sub groups. We have found sub classification a useful but not absolute prognostic index. This accords with the views of Bosch, Stauffer and Nickel

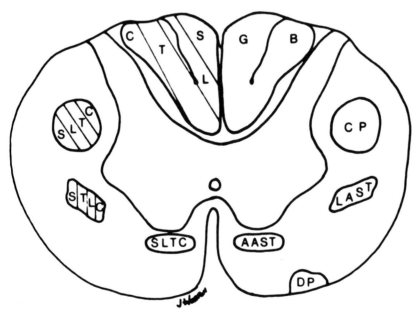

Figure 4.7. Diagrammatic cross section of spinal cord at C6. G fasciculus gracilis (Goll) 'sensory' for lower extremities and lumbar region; B fasciculus cuneatus (Burdach) 'sensory' for thoracic region and upper extremities; CP crossed pyramidal (lateral corticospinal) voluntary muscle; DP direct pyramidal (anterior corticospinal) voluntary muscle. Neck, upper limbs; LAST lateral ascending spinothalamic. Pain and temperature. Some touch?; AAST anterior ascending spinothalamic. Light touch; C cervical; T thoracic; L lumbar; S sacral; ('sensory' = joint position sense, two point discrimination, deep touch and pressure. Vibration).

(1971), Braakman and Penning (1971) and Marar (1974).

There are five main groups. To understand these syndromes some knowledge of the gross anatomy of the spinal tracts is necessary (Figure 4.7).

i Incomplete lesions

Incomplete lesions (sub-total syndrome) with partial preservation of motor and sensory function below the level of injury have a good prognosis. Rapid improvement during the first week offers hope of recovery to normal or near normal.

ii Anterior cord syndromes

Here there is complete motor paralysis below the level of injury with some blunting of sensation and loss of pain and temperature appreciation, but sparing of deep pressure sensation, two point discrimination, joint position sense and vibration.

Schneider (1955) attributes this syndrome to compression or destruction of the anterior part of the cord. A similar picture may be seen in thrombosis of the anterior spinal artery, but this is a phenomenon rarely seen in spinal cord injuries. The prognosis is poor.

iii Posterior cord syndrome

There is no loss of muscle power or thermal discrimination. The impairment in the posterior column function is evident by loss of deep pressure sensation, deep pain and proprioception. Variations from the pure form, for example more widespread sensory loss with painful symptoms referred to the shoulder girdles and upper limbs, are common. The prognosis is good but the patient is left with some degree of ataxia which may be very disabling. The syndrome may be encountered in every type of spinal injury, but is most often seen in hyperextension injuries with fractures of the posterior elements, and in the rare direct injury of the neural arch.

iv Brown-Sequard syndrome

The greater motor loss and the impairment of joint position sense, two point discrimination sense and vibration are on the side of the injury. There is loss of pain and temperature appreciation on the opposite side of the body with minimal motor loss. The prognosis for sphincter control and walking (although often with a below knee orthosis) is good.

The impairment of pain and thermal discrimination in the limbs showing the greater motor recovery is commonly permanent. This syndrome is most often encountered in stab wounds and in fractures of the lateral masses, but is not uncommon in high cervical injuries.

v Central cord syndrome

This is seen classically in hyperextension injuries of the spondylotic spines of older patients. It may however occur in any type of cervical injury, and it is the commonest of the incomplete cord syndromes. It is caused by haemorrhage into the central grey matter with a varying degree of white matter involvement (Figure 4.8). The clinical picture varies in severity, but is normally worse in upper than lower limbs. It is characterized by a flaccid lower motor neurone paralysis of the hands and arms and a spastic upper motor neurone paresis of the legs. The sensory fibres for the trunk and lower limbs are usually spared, but there is commonly some impairment of sphincter function. The prognosis, as with all neurological injuries, is better in younger patients. In older patients recovery of finger function is poor and often made worse by the development of joint stiffness. The ability to walk improves slowly but is hampered often by spasticity.

When the neurological and radiological findings do not agree, further radiographic studies may be indicated. These may demonstrate vertebral injuries at other levels (Bentley and McSweeney, 1968). The discrepancy between the vertebral levels and the neurological segments must be taken into account, as must the occasional temporary ascent of the lesion, and the longitudinal nature of some cord injuries.

Radiography

'X-rays show the resting position and not the dynamics of the injury.' (A.G. Hardy.)

The initial X-ray examination is often incomplete and not infrequently fails to

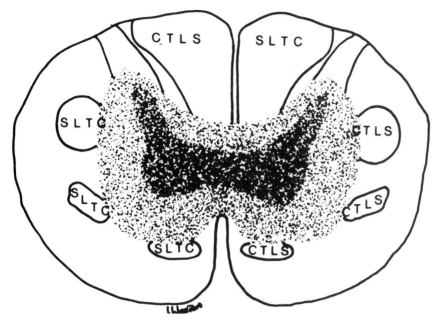

Figure 4.8. Diagram to show central cord syndrome: darker areas of spreading haemorrhage involve C (cervical) more than L (lumbar) or S (sacral).

include the seventh cervical vertebral body. This is one of the commonest errors and has led to many medico-legal problems following missed lower cervical dislocations. The lower part of the cervical spine is overshadowed by the shoulders which are often elevated by muscle spasm. Long axis traction on the extended arms may help to display C7. Abduction elevation of the arm with the opposite shoulder depressed (swimmer's view) and the beam at a 60° angle is often useful and in cases of doubt lateral tomograms may be helpful. High quality anteroposterior projections should be studied for abnormalities of the lateral masses and spinous process alignment, as deviation of a spinous process may indicate unilateral facet dislocation, while approximation of processes may be seen in bilateral dislocations. A good quality open mouth view is essential also for the atlanto-axial region. In the lateral view widening of the interval between the spinous processes may indicate a severe flexion injury, while backwards displacement suggests a hyperextension force.

More precise examination requires the presence of the radiologist and the surgeon together with the radiographer. We have

found that the 45° supine oblique views display the intervertebral foramina and the line of the apophyseal joints to the cervicothoracic junction (McCall, Park and McSweeney, 1973). In this projection there is no need to move the patient's neck (Figure 4.9). In young children whose spines are naturally hypermobile there is often great difficulty in interpreting the X-rays with reference to the presence or absence of abnormal motion (Figure 4.10).

The precise history of the injury is important in evaluating the degree of trauma. The presence of a retropharyngeal soft tissue shadow and failure to correct a subluxation when the spine is gently extended are confirmatory signs of injury. Excellent accounts of paediatric radiography are available in the writings of Cattell and Filtzer (1965), Von Torklus and Gehle (1972), Fielding (1973) and Silverman and Kattan (1975). Conventional and computed tomography have been shown to be of equal value in defining the extent of bone and joint injury (Clark *et al.*, 1988). While lateral tomography is most helpful for the facet joints below C2, CT scanning is of more value for the posterior elements and upper cervical spine. (Figure 4.11a,b).

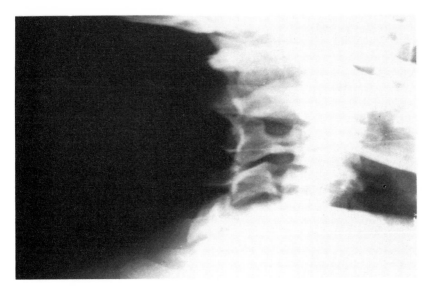

Figure 4.9. Dislocation right facet C4,5. Supine oblique view.

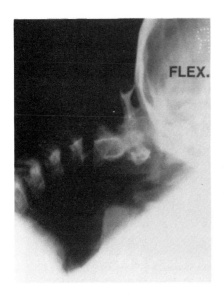
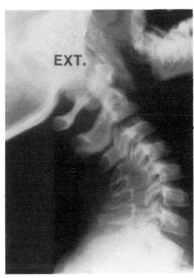

Figure 4.10. Soft tissue neck injury in a child. No neurological deficit. Is there instability at C2/3? (See Figure 4.24).

There is no place for discography in the acute injury and in our view myelography is very rarely indicated and may result in dramatic neurological deterioration. MRI scanning, while providing details of soft tissue (disc and cord) damage is not only of limited availability, but also difficult to employ in a seriously ill and recently injured patient.

In general, the correct and careful application of conventional plain radiology including oblique views and tomography will provide all the information necessary to manage the patient, but will require the close cooperation and consultation of surgeon, radiologist and radiographer.

Radiological classification

The neurological classification described earlier is unquestionably a better guide to functional recovery than are inferences from

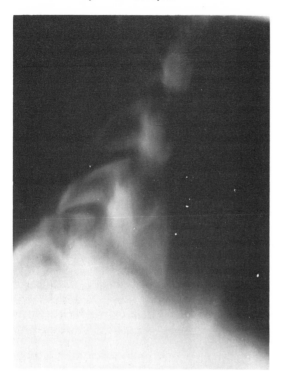

Figure 4.11. (a) Facet fracture seen on lateral tomography. (b) Fracture arch of atlas (CT scan).

a

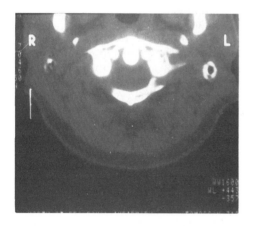
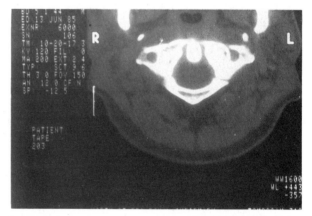
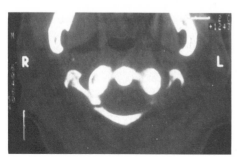
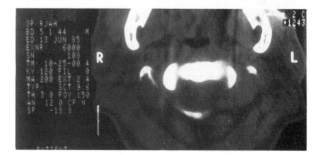

b

the initial radiographs. In practice, however, it is important to be familiar with and recognize the implications of the X-ray appearances which offer both a guide to immediate treatment and an indication of predicted long-term stability.

The majority of injuries will fall into four main groups. These are: 1 flexion, 2 compression, 3 hyperextension, and 4 a miscellaneous group.

It must be appreciated that 'pure' flexion and hyperextension injuries are uncommon, and that rotation, shearing, and less commonly lateral bending forces, are a part of the mechanism. Compression is a common component of injury to the spine and its use as a descriptive term is hallowed in the radiological and clinical literature. The opposite force of distraction is uncommon but may occur as in one type of hangman's fracture or as a result of injudicious skull traction (Figure 4.12). The addition of a shearing element in certain circumstances will produce dislocations as shown by Bauze and Ardran (1978).

For detailed descriptions of the fundamental work the important papers of Barnes (1948), Taylor and Blackwood (1948), Taylor (1951), Schneider, Cherry and Pantek (1954), Whitley and Forsyth (1960), Roaf (1960, 1972), Holdsworth (1963), Forsyth (1964), Cornish (1968) and Selecki and Williams (1970) should be consulted. More recently, useful classifica-

tions have been described by Gehweiler, Osborne and Becker (1980) and Harris, Edeiken-Monroe and Kopaniky (1986), the latter employing the two column concept described by White and Panjabi (1978).

1 Flexion (hyperanteflexion)

Pure flexion forces are restrained by the posterior ligament complex (mainly the capsules of the facet joints, ligamentum flavum and the interspinous ligament), the posterior neck muscles and the impact of the chin on the sternum. These forces may result in relatively minor compression fractures of the vertebral body, and the ligament complex may remain intact. When flexion force is greater, the impact of the chin on the sternum may act as a fulcrum so that with continuation of the force an anterior maginal fracture is produced. Such injuries are seldom accompanied by neurological impairment.

When a rotational force is added ligament rupture occurs and permits a unilateral facet dislocation which may lock in the displaced position. Forces of greater magnitude will produce a bilateral dislocation leaving only the anterior longitudinal ligament intact. Lesser degrees of force which do not completely disrupt the capsular ligaments may cause a 'dimple' fracture of the vertebral body and a

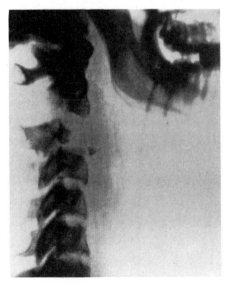

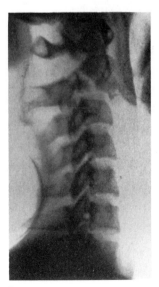

Figure 4.12. (a) Over distraction of hangman's fracture by excessive traction. (b) After reduction of weight. Uneventful healing. No neurology.

a   b

partial subluxation of the facet joints. We have called this the 'hidden flexion injury' (Webb *et al.*, 1976) and similar cases have been reported by Stringa (1964), Cheshire (1969) and Evans (1976).

The associated posterior ligament disruption may lead to progressive kyphotic deformity and increasing joint subluxation. If such an injury is suspected flexion extension lateral films may be helpful. These should be carried out under sedation and under medical supervision. Even then muscle spasm may mask the injury and if necessary the films should be repeated in a few days when the spasm has subsided. Recognition of injuries of this type which may lead to anterior subluxation is important if later neurological deterioration and late deformity is to be prevented (Figure 4.13a,b).

Lateral flexion injuries per se are uncommon (Roaf, 1963) and result in fractures of the facet, transverse process, or merely a slight separation of the vertebral bodies on the side of injury. There may be an accompanying branchial plexus lesion, and cord damage, if present, is often complete.

2 Compression (axial loading)

Compression fractures may produce wedging or comminution of the vertebral body whether the head is flexed or extended. The posterior ligament complex is usually intact. The X-ray appearances vary. There may be indentation of the vertebral body on its anterosuperior surface, or there may be separation of a large anteroinferior marginal fragment as in one

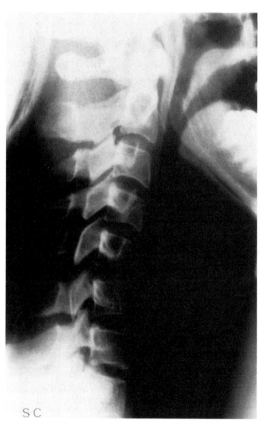
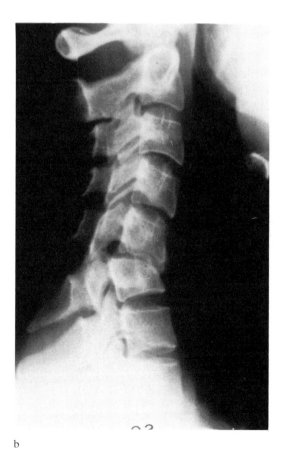

a   b

Figure 4.13. (a) Flexion injury with posterior ligament disruption and joint subluxation. Significant tetraparesis. (b) As (a) after conservative treatment. Spontaneous fusion with kyphotic deformity. Asymptomatic. Full neurological recovery.

variety of 'teardrop' fracture (see Figure 4.1). The significance of this severe injury is that the remainder of the vertebral body and disc is pushed backwards into the spinal canal (Schneider and Kahn, 1956). In another type the X-rays suggest an 'explosive' effect with loss of depth and lateral spread of the vertebral body. This is accompanied by the retropulsion of bone against the anterior aspect of the cord (Holdsworth, 1965). The neurological loss if often severe with tetraplegia or anterior cord syndrome.

3 Hyperextension (hyperdeflexion; retroflexion)

We are greatly indebted to Whitley and Forsyth (1960) and Forsyth (1964) for their analysis and definition of these injuries. As the head and neck are forced into hyperextension the posterior elements are so crowded together as to fracture the facets, and these acting as a fulcrum cause rupture of the anterior longitudinal ligament. They point out that as the force continues, the head moves through an arc travelling backwards and downwards. If allowed to continue it will finally be travelling in a forward direction. As the cervical spine travels forwards, the forces are transmitted to the facet joints and posterior elements, resulting in compression fractures, and ultimately anterior ligament rupture. This is brought about when facet joint fracture permits the continuing force to push the vertebral body forwards. It finally comes to rest in a position of anterior displacement (Figure 4.14a,b). Unless the circumstances of the injury, the presence of

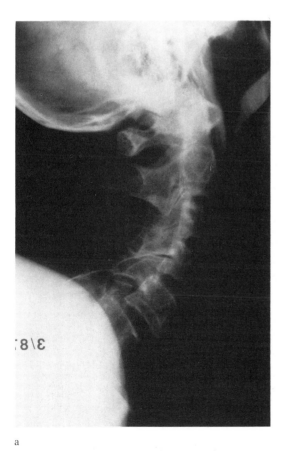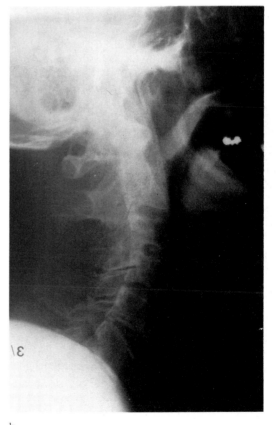

a b

Figure 4.14. (a) Hyperextension injury C5,6 ending in anterior displacement of body of C5. (b) Same patient as (a) after reduction. Note hyperextension at level of injury.

frontal bruising, and the features of the X-rays are analysed, the forward displacement of the body may be mistaken for a flexion injury. This led Burke (1971) to describe the final stage of this injury as 'masquerading' as one of flexion. In this severe form of hyperextension injury with forward displacement of the vertebral body there is usually an antero-inferior chip fracture of the displaced body.

Other suspicious signs are fractures of the laminae, pedicles and a fracture near the base of the spinous process, all of which tend to be displaced upwards. In addition there is evidence of displacement or compression of the inferior articular process of the displaced body ('horizontal facet'). This is in contrast to flexion injuries when the superior facet of the vertebra below may be fractured. The injury is unstable and attempts at reduction with skull calipers may fail.

Other patterns of injury are seen when the static X-rays in the neutral position show little or no displacement of the vertebral body. There may be tell-tale chip fractures of the antero-inferior margin of the upper vertebra, or a similar fragment avulsed from the antero-superior surface of the body below. These indicate damage to the anterior longitudinal ligament.

All grades of severity occur from extensive disruptions of both longitudinal ligaments to cases in which no bony or ligament injury can be demonstrated.

The latter include many elderly patients in whom spondylosis of the cervical spine (often with an upper dorsal kyphosis) is common. Post-mortem studies not infrequently reveal anterior longitudinal ligament rupture and one or more disc disruptions (Kinoshita and Hirakawa, 1989).

The neurological picture and potential for recovery vary considerably. In some the neural impairment is so slight as to suggest a concussion effect on the microcirculation of the cord (Hughes and Brownwell, 1963). In others the 'pincer' action of the ligamentum flavum and posterior osteophytes (the Taylor and Black-wood mechanism) is reflected in the more extensive paralysis and a poorer recovery. The radiological signs in these patients may include anterior widening of the disc space with closure when the disc is immobilized in flexion.

Special vigilance is essential in the suspected hyperextension injury of younger patients

when the X-rays show no vertebral body displacement. The adjacent disc spaces should be compared, and minor flake fractures or alteration in alignment should arouse suspicion.*

A traction film – that is a lateral X-ray after the application of 13.6–16 kg (30–35 lb) weight – may better demonstrate disruption and more safely than flexion extension films in such cases (Stauffer, 1984, personal communication).

Occasionally the superior vertebral body may be displaced backwards (Figure 4.15). In one of our cases there was an associated fracture of the hyoid bone and the patient died within an hour of admission to hospital. Almost complete severance of the cord was noted at post mortem. Burke (1971) mentions a comparable case.

4 Miscellaneous

This group includes direct injuries with compound wounds, congenital anomalies (Figure 4.16), and fracture dislocation with pre-existing pathology, notably rheumatoid arthritis and ankylosing spondylitis.

Treatment

1 General considerations

As with dorsal and lumbar injuries, so with cervical injuries, there has been, is, and for the foreseeable future will be a continuing debate on the relative merits of operative and conservative treatment, of different types of orthoses, and of the options of medical management.

---

*Extension of the neck has been postulated as a cause of sudden death in infancy. It was invoked also by Sir Frederic Treves as the cause of death in the Elephant Man. To quote the *British Medical Journal* of 1890: 'The Elephant Man's head had apparently grown so heavy that he had difficulty in holding it up and had to sleep in a sitting and crouching position with his hands clasped over his legs and his head on his knees. If he lay down flat the heavy head tended to fall back and produce a feeling of suffocation. He was found dead by the ward maid lying across his bed. Mr Treves was of the opinion that the "ponderous skull had fallen backwards and dislocated his neck." The Coroner, however, felt that the Elephant Man's windpipe had been compressed by the heavy head causing asphyxia'. (Vanezis, 1989)

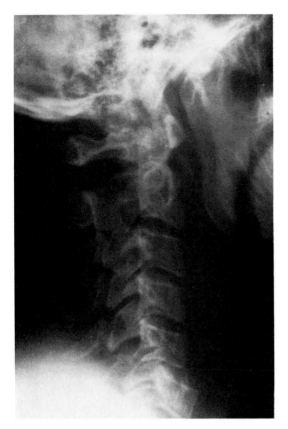

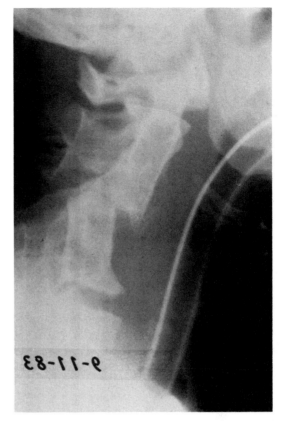

Figure 4.15. Dislocation C5,6. Posterior displacement body of C5. Probable hyperextension injury. Complete tetraplegia.

Figure 4.16. Fracture dislocation in Klippel–Feil syndrome. Initially undiagnosed. Late onset tetraplegia.

The issues are multifactorial, and the decisions taken frequently result from the likely long-term effect on the patient.

A tetraplegic in the UK will be in the same total care unit for 9–12 months until rehabilitation is complete and he or she is resettled. Under such circumstances operation to permit mobilization a few weeks earlier has little to offer. In North America, on the other hand, such surgery may permit early transfer from a high to a low dependency unit, representing an important financial saving. By the same token, British patients given the choice, tend to opt for non-operative treatment, while one's impression is that North American patients (and their relatives) are more likely to demand that 'something must be done'.

In less developed countries, by contrast, there may be no question of choice as the facilities for intensive care and sophisticated spinal surgery are commonly unavailable.

Decisions concerning treatment will vary therefore from place to place and from unit to unit, for a variety of very good reasons, including, in particular, the presence or absence of neurological deficit. Somewhat disappointingly perhaps, it remains a matter of fact, that in the great majority of cases the long-term outcome will be the same whatever the line of management, provided it is competent. Even the reduction of gross displacement such as bilateral facet dislocation does not appear to influence the long-term result either from the point of view of the cord or spinal column function (Dall, 1972).

What must be taken into account of course are the age and physical state of the patient, and an aggressive surgical approach which may be appropriate for a young healthy person may be most inappropriate for the elderly, infirm or severely paralysed with respiratory and metabolic problems. The remarkable improvement in the survival of patients with severe neurological impairment in recent years is due more to improved medical care, early and late, than to advances in surgical technique. The philosophy of long-term management heralded by the pioneer work of Guttmann (1973), Munro (1952), and others has completely changed the prospects of the severely paralysed. In this account therefore an eclectic approach is advocated, to be based on the patient's general condition, the surgeon's experience and the quality of ancillary care available.

2   Injuries with associated cord damage

Dislocations and fracture dislocations should be reduced as a matter of urgency by skull traction, manipulation or open reduction, and gross misalignment from fracture corrected by traction in recumbency. The first few hours after injury are crucial and every effort must be made to realign the spinal column quickly and safely in order to provide the damaged cord with the best chance of recovery and to protect it from further injury. While there are many cases where a dislocation left unreduced has fused spontaneously and led to no further harm, one has seen patients where tetraplegia undoubtedly has not occurred until some hours after an undiagnosed and unreduced dislocation, while there are reported cases where early reduction appears to have led to recovery of a complete lesion (Duke, 1981). Traction or manipulation under anaesthesia is usually successful in achieving reduction and open reduction as an emergency is seldom indicated. Such an operation risks further damage to an already damaged and unstable spinal cord. While some authors favour early anterior decompression of burst fractures, this has not been proven to be of value in assisting neurological recovery. On the other hand, a high mortality for acute surgery in patients with complete tetraplegia together with possibly impaired neurological recovery in incomplete lesions following early anterior operation has been reported recently from Australia (Osti, Fraser and Griffiths, 1989). The evidence is that for patients with neurological impairment open operation is better carried out as a late planned elective procedure when the condition of patient and cord have stabilized.

3   Injuries without cord damage

Early reduction of dislocations is advisable but not essential. Whether or not this is carried out, conservative treatment with skull traction may be instituted while the full extent of the injury is assessed and the patient is given the opportunity to consider the alternatives of operative or conservative long-term treatment. If the patient is seen after a week or more with an unreduced dislocation, conservative treatment is strongly recommended and open correction at that time is fraught with danger (Ramadier and Bombart, 1964).

We have seen in medico-legal practice a number of disasters when late reduction of a 'missed fracture dislocation' has been carried out. Having said that, it must be pointed out that Verbiest (1962, 1973) has reported good results from anterior or anterolateral correction in cases of many months' duration.

4   Early progression of an incomplete lesion

This is an uncommon occurrence in cervical injuries and must be distinguished from the rise of one or two segments sometimes encountered in patients with a complete cord lesion. Ascent of the lesion then is usually attributed to oedema and recovery takes place gradually over the next few days. Rarely, the permanent loss of several segments may result from cord infarction.

Other causes of neurological deterioration are excessive traction and increasing local displacement when the nature of the injury has not been recognized, for example when an extension injury is mistaken for one of flexion (Figure 4.17). We have seen a number of patients develop increasing neurological deficit after being allowed to sit up prematurely. This phenomenon of neurological instability is attributable to cord hypoxia from hypotension, it is seen in upper dorsal lesions also, and is a further argument against rapid early mobilization (Baker, 1984, personal communication).

Assuming other causes have been excluded, the remote possibility of an extradural spinal haematoma or other unexpected lesions must be considered, and a CT scan may be helpful.

This is a convenient place to mention that routine laminectomy has nothing to offer in

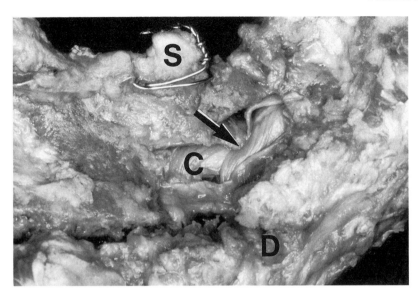

Figure 4.17. Late neurological deterioration in hyperextension dislocation following posterior fusion. Note edge of lamina indenting cord. (Arrow). S = spinous process. C = cord. D = disrupted disc. (Same patient as Figure 4.14.)

the management of these patients. As previously practised it created not infrequently the problem of progressive deformity. It still has a place in the management of open wounds and rarely in posterior pressure on the cord by depressed laminae.

Treatment of spinal cord injuries

1 General principles

When the spinal injury is complicated by cord damage the effects on other systems are widespread. In cervical injuries, motor, sensory and autonomic dysfunction leads to cardiorespiratory, gastrointestinal and renal problems, with impairment of sphincter control. Only a limited discussion on the more important problems is appropriate here. For more detailed information the reader is referred to the works of Guttmann (1973), Hardy and Rossier (1975), Pierce and Nickel (1977), and Bedbrook (1981).

2 Respiratory problems

Pulmonary insufficiency with vital capacities of under a litre requires frequent 'chesting' and assisted respiration by a competent physio-

therapist. All staff and relatives should be familiar with these procedures and assist in them.

In patients with chronic chest disease or associated chest injury a mini tracheostomy may be very helpful in permitting tracheal toilet and avoiding intubation. Formal tracheostomy has special risks in these patients (Frankel, 1970), may be difficult to reverse later, and should be avoided if possible.

The recording of the breathing pattern is an essential part of the nursing records and repeated blood gas analyses and vital capacity measurements are essential if there is any doubt about respiratory function. With these measures we are able to avoid tracheostomy in all but a few of our patients.

It is important to be aware of overloading the labile cardiovascular system and intravenous fluid should be used with caution.

3 Gastrointestinal care

The complication of paralytic ileus can usually be averted by early passage of a nasal gastric tube. Solid food should be withheld until bowel sounds are present, and oral fluids introduced slowly. Abdominal distension adds to the respiratory embarrassment and the passage of a flatus tube may be helpful.

Routine medication with histamine antagonists should be commenced early as peptic ulceration and gastrointestinal bleeding are common complications.

4 Care of the bladder

The general adoption of aseptic intermittent catheterization has brought about a great improvement in the management of patients who have suffered spinal cord injury. Unless the bladder is distended there is normally no urgency to pass a catheter in the first 24 hours, during which stage renal suppression is common. The initial catheterization in a male should be done by one of the medical staff. In our unit subsequent catheterization is carried out by trained orderlies or senior nursing staff. Fluid intake is carefully monitored and the bladder must not be permitted to over-distend. This regimen has revolutionized the management of the paralysed bladder. An automatic pattern of micturition can be anticipated within a few weeks of injury.

The passage of a wide bore balloon catheter in the receiving hospital is condemned as it will lead to infection and urethral trauma, and militates against the adoption of the intermittent regimen. Meticulous attention to detail and particularly asepsis is required (Guttmann and Frankel, 1966; Walsh, 1968; Pearman and England, 1973).

5 Thromboembolism

Anticoagulants should be commenced as soon as it is safe to do so as there is a high incidence of thromboembolism, not infrequently fatal in these patients.

6 The timing of operative interference

Minor surgical procedures, including manipulation under general anaesthesia, can be carried out with reasonable safety at any time. Where there are multiple injuries, essential major operations should be performed within 24 hours, if possible, before respiratory problems and metabolic imbalance supervene. On the other hand, it is usually wiser to defer non-urgent major surgery for 10 days or so, by

which time the patient's general condition should be stable.

7 Beds

An ordinary hospital bed with an outrigger to support the traction pulley is satisfactory, provided a 2-hourly turning regimen is instituted in the paralysed patient. This may be carried out safely on a conventional bed by an experienced team, and should be commenced on admission. However, a variety of mechanical turning beds are available, and at least one should be available in every District Hospital.

8 Spinal Injury Unit

When serious neurological injury has occurred, early transfer to a specialized unit is imperative. Much will depend on local circumstances and the proximity of such a centre, but the advantages of a competent nursing and respiratory team, and experienced overall care, leading to optimal functional, social, and vocational rehabilitation such a service provides need no emphasis.

9 Application of skull traction

Serious cervical injuries will require the application of skull traction, which in fact is a misnomer. Although traction is used in reduction, what is meant by maintenance traction is rather external skeletal stabilization seldom exceeding 2.3 or 2.7 kg (5 or 6 lb) in weight. A halter should never be used in the treatment of acute spinal injuries. Complications such as submental pressure sore or jugular thrombosis have been reported (Baker, 1984, personal communication). If a halo vest will be employed later, halo traction may be instituted. More often skull calipers will be used. A number of different devices are available (Figure 4.18).

Credit is due to Crutchfield (1938) for his innovation, but his calipers are now outmoded. They are clumsy to insert and fall out readily. Gardner-Wells calipers have many advantages, including the fact that the instructions for their insertion are attached to them. They have the disadvantage that they project widely to the

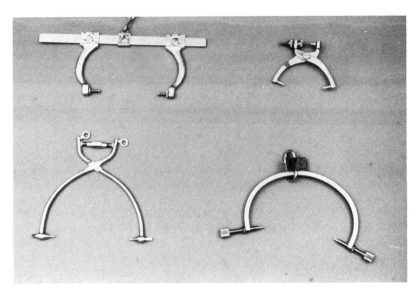

Figure 4.18. Skull calipers. Clockwise from top left: Blackburn's Crutchfield's, Gardner-Wells, Cone's (D.J. Grundy with permission).

side of the head, interfering with nursing, and some therefore prefer Cone's. Blackburn's penetrate the skull readily and are dangerous for that reason.

Once applied calipers should be pain free. They must be inspected daily and adjusted as necessary. Complications such as CSF leak and extradural abscess occur rarely and some have been described by Weisl (1972). The most common complication however is dislodgement of the pin from the bone, converting skull to scalp traction. This is easily overlooked and should be suspected if the patient complains of pain.

Treatment of spinal column injury

A Upper cervical spine (occiput to C3)

As the canal diameter above the third cervical vertebra is twice that of the cord, skeletal injuries at this level, even with quite gross displacement, are commonly unassociated with cord damage. When the latter does occur, it is frequently incomplete, and often of Brown-Sequard type. Improved resuscitation techniques and 'flying squads' have led, however, to the survival of the small but increasing number of complete high cord lesions, ventilator dependent, posing major social and economic long-term problems.

Patients with upper cervical injury commonly complain only of neck and occipital pain or neuralgia. Interpretation of the X-rays may be difficult, and the commonly occurring congenital anomalies in the area may add to the difficulty. The shadow of a prevertebral haematoma may be an important clue, and the back of the throat should be inspected for this phenomenon also.

A i Atlanto-occipital dislocation

While occipitocervical injuries may be very common (Davis *et al.*, 1973), most are fatal, and only a small number of survivors of atlanto-occipital dislocation with neurological recovery have been reported. In the case reported by Gabrielson and Maxwell (1966), there was massive swelling of the posterior part of the neck with the sixth nerve palsy. The injury was not apparent until skull traction was applied. Evarts' (1970) case had a hemiparesis which improved on traction. Diffuse spasticity was noticed by Page *et al.* (1973). The patient described by Eismont and Bohlman (1978) had a spastic tetraparesis more marked in the upper limbs which gradually resolved, although the blood pressure remained labile for many weeks. The neurological picture resembled the cruciate paralyses described by Bell (1976) in lesions compressing the upper portion of the pyramidal decussation.

In these cases, once the patient's condition permits, posterior occipitocervical fusion is the treatment of choice.

A ii Fractures of the atlas

It is a curious feature of cervical injuries that, in general, the less the clinical significance of a lesion the greater the volume of literature devoted to it. Certainly this is true of odontoid fractures and to a lesser extent it applies to injuries of the atlas. However, in this case, the literature is not only extensive, but of considerable historic interest, commencing with Sir Geoffrey Jefferson's paper* (1920) and subsequent Hunterian lecture (1924) (McSweeney, 1980, first edition of this book).

Sir Geoffrey's description of a four part fracture has been challenged more recently by Hays and Alker (1988) on the basis that it has not proved possible to create such an injury experimentally or to demonstrate it. However, Levine and Edwards (1986) provide radiographic proof of just such an injury. In any event, the principle of the burst fracture with separation at times of the lateral masses remains true.

Lateral mass fracture as an isolated injury requires symptomatic treatment only. Two distinct patterns of injury to the ring of the atlas occur. The more minor is the posterior arch fracture resulting from a hyperextension force and commonly associated with injury to the odontoid. As an isolated injury the posterior arch fracture requires symptomatic treatment only (see Figure 4.11b).

*Sir Geoffrey Jefferson recounts the following story which he culled from Jean Lewis Petit's *Maladies des os.* 'The six or seven year old son of a work man went into the shop of a neighbour, a friend of the father. In playing with the child he put one of his hands under the chin, the other behind the head and lifted him up in the air "to show him his grandfather" a vulgar saying.
No sooner had the child left the ground than he resisted, dislocated his neck and died on the spot. His father, told immediately what had happened, was transported with rage, ran after his neighbour and being unable to overtake him, he threw a saddler's hammer which he happened to have in his hand. The sharp end pierced the muscles in what is called the pit of the neck. Cutting all the muscles it penetrated the space between the 1st and 2nd vertebrae of the neck, it cut the spinal cord and caused his instant death. Thus these two deaths came in almost the same fashion'. Sir Geoffrey goes on to say that the tale may have been traditional two hundred years ago, but apparently Petit did not state whether the story had been given him by an eye witness!

The second pattern, the true burst fracture results from a vertical compression force, and is associated with damage to the front and back of the ring. Spence, Decker and Sell (1970) on the basis of one clinical case and some experimental work concluded that separation of the lateral masses by more than 6.9 mm indicates rupture of the transverse ligament and constitutes an indication for surgical fusion. Sherk and Nicholson (1970) and Landells and Van Peteghem (1988) concluded however that simple conservative treatment was appropriate for all atlantal fractures and this is our view also. While Levine and Edwards (1986) recommended halo traction for 6–8 weeks in an attempt to achieve some reduction of widely displaced lateral masses, this is not our practice. We advocate light traction for 2 or 3 weeks until spasm and pain have subsided, followed by mobilization in a collar for the less displaced injury, and a Minerva cast for those deemed potentially unstable.

A iii Rupture of the transverse ligament of the atlas

As an isolated injury this leads to increased atlanto-axial displacement in flexion and commonly is diagnosed late. If the diagnosis is made early ambulant treatment in a rigid orthosis may result in sufficient soft tissue healing to restore stability. When the condition is diagnosed late, atlanto-axial fusion should be offered if it is symptomatic or if the degree of movement exceeds 5–7 mm or shows signs of progression. The same advice applies when early conservative management fails to resolve instability. Levine and Edwards (1986) hold the opposite view and believe primary posterior fusion to be the treatment of choice in all cases.

A iv Atlanto-axial rotary abnormalities

Although the word 'rotatory' is commonly applied to these injuries, 'rotary' or 'rotative' are more correct, meaning as they do 'caused by rotation', while rotatory is defined as 'connected with, working by means of, or causing rotations'.

Problems of atlanto-axial rotary displacement form a curious group of incompletely understood conditions, all characterized by the

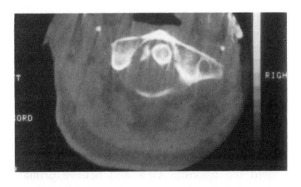

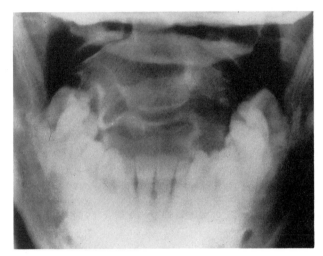

Figure 4.19. (a) Acute unilateral traumatic rotary dislocation of C1,2 in an adult, lateral view. (b) Open mouth view. (c) CT scan.

a

b

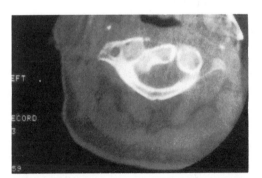

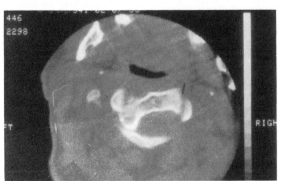

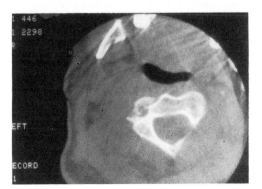

c

'Cock Robin' position of the head and radiological subluxation or dislocation of at least one atlanto-axial joint. Pain is not a prominent feature and neurological problems are rare (Corner, 1907).

At one end of the spectrum there exists the condition of true dislocation. We have seen one late case in an adult (Figure 4.19a,b and c). Left untreated, his head position improved as the lower cervical spine compensated, his injury was stable, and he was left with significant loss of neck movement but no other symptoms. If the condition is diagnosed early, manipulation under general (or local, Levine and Edwards, 1986) anaesthetic would seem a reasonable option if the dislocation will not reduce on traction (Jackson, 1927; Greeley, 1930).

At the opposite end of the spectrum are those cases which are not traumatic in origin – rotary subluxation in children associated with upper respiratory tract infections. These problems resolve spontaneously.

A patient who had apparently developed a facility to dislocate his atlanto-axial joint at will was described by Brav (1936). Seeking admission to hospital after various accidents this patient was later arrested for obtaining money on false pretenses. Haralson and Boyd (1969) reported on an inebriated patient, the victim of a road traffic accident, who suffered a posterior dislocation of the atlas without fracture of the odontoid process. Reduction was secured by manual traction with rotation and forward pressure on the occiput. The dislocation was reduced with an audible snap.

In between these extremes is a group of children who present with the condition apparently as a result of trauma, but often developing 2 or 3 weeks later (Figure 4.20). Not uncommonly such children confuse the issue by having a cold as well! The radiological diagnosis is confused by the fact that it is not possible to tell if any abnormality seen is pathological or purely postural. Fortunately,

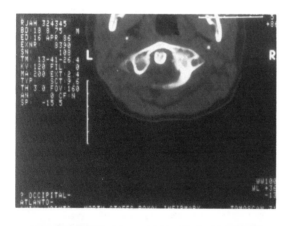
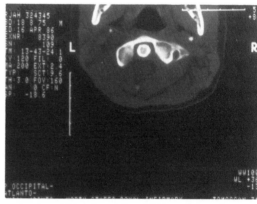
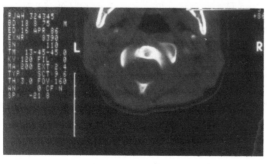
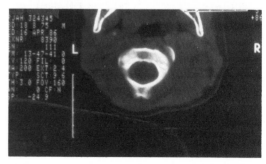

Figure 4.20. Unilateral post-traumatic C1,2 rotary dislocation in a child. Spontaneous resolution.

the majority of such cases resolve quickly and completely with a short period of halter traction and a soft collar, and late instability is rare (Birney and Hanley, 1989). We have seen one curious case of onset 1–2 weeks after a road traffic accident which resulted in significant facial injuries, where the deformity reversed from one side to the other over night while on halter traction. Examination under anaesthetic revealed a full range of normal movement and no apparent abnormality, and the child woke up from the anaesthetic cured! Occasionally however late instability or fixed deformity may result and require surgical attention (Phillips and Hensinger, 1989).

A v Fracture of the odontoid process of the axis

'We ask your consideration of fractures of the odontoid process. . . First, because the rarity of their occurrence is in inverse ratio to the gravity of their symptoms. . . Second, because an early recognition of the lesion may save life and make possible the pursuit of happiness. . .' (Osgood and Lund, 1928).

Since this was written, the hazards of fracture of the odontoid have come to be regarded with less gravity, for at that time the mortality of the condition was believed to be more than 50 per cent. That this is not the case has been demonstrated by a number of authors. Pringle (1974) in a retrospective study of 62 cases recorded nine deaths in elderly patients within 3 months of injury, but in only one was the fracture a possible cause of death, while six of the other eight were proven at post mortem to be from unrelated causes.

The well known classification of Anderson and D'Alonzo (1974) has proved helpful in the management of these injuries and accords well with clinical experience. Taken as a group they represent some 10 per cent of all cervical fractures and despite often alarming displacement are infrequently associated with spinal cord injury (5/62 in Pringle's series).

The mechanism of injury is complex and variable, consisting of flexion or extension, often with an element of compression or rotation, and sometimes shear (Selecki and Williams, 1970). To some extent the position of the head and mandible at the moment of impact dictate the outcome. There is an incidence of up to 10 per cent of coexistent

dorsal spine fracture, and associated head injuries, often minor, are virtually universal.

In between 10 and 40 per cent of cases conservative treatment results in non-union, and while in the majority this is of doubtful clinical significance, occasional reports of late myelopathy (Elliot and Sachs, 1912; Khan and Yglesias, 1935; Askenasy, Braham and Kosary, 1960; Wadia, 1967) lead some to advocate posterior fusion as a routine in such cases.

Tomography may be helpful both in diagnosis and in ascertaining the degree of union (Nachemson, 1960).

Type I fractures are uncommon, often of rotational nature, and require symptomatic treatment only (Figure 4.21a).

The majority of type II fractures (Figure 4.21b) are undisplaced or displaced posteriorly, and result from hyperextension injury to elderly patients who fall. There is a high incidence of associated cervical spondylosis, which may, by its rigidity, contribute to the fracture and the subsequent non-union, and may lead also to an accompanying central cord syndrome.

This last is often attributed mistakenly to the fracture itself. The non-union rate of some 40 per cent has led to the advocacy of a halo vest (Levine and Edwards, 1986) or routine posterior fusion (Clark and White, 1985) as primary treatment. The former has significant complications and is poorly tolerated by the older patient, while primary fusion is inexcusably radical. We agree with Pepin, Bourne and Hawkins (1981) that 'an aggressive attempt to obtain union is not the treatment of choice in the elderly' and advocate symptomatic treatment in that age group and a halo vest or Minerva cast in the young.

Type III fractures (Figure 4.21c) more commonly are the result of road traffic accidents to younger people, take the form of flexion injuries, and tend towards anterior displacement. They may be managed by postural reduction and immobilization in halo vest or Minerva, and the majority unite. However, Clark and White (1985) reported that they may not be as benign as previously thought, and felt surgery might be indicated for 'unstable' injuries of this type. This is not our experience.

The management of established non-union must take into account the type of patient, the symptoms, and the degree of instability

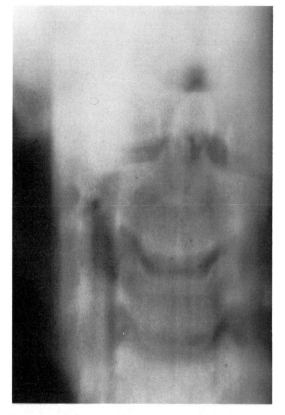

a

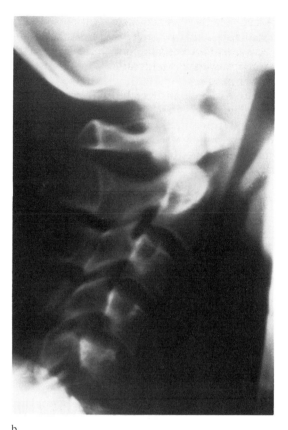

b

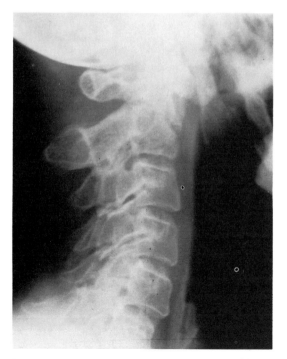

c

Figure 4.21. (a) Odontoid fracture type I. (b) Odontoid fracture type II. (c) Odontoid fracture type III.

present. In the elderly, and those without symptoms and/or instability, the pros and cons of fusion should be discussed, but the condition may be best left untreated and kept under long-term review.

There would appear to be no more indication for surgery for such cases than there is for an asymptomatic os odontoideum diagnosed by chance. For symptomatic instability, particularly in the younger age group, atlanto-axial fusion is the treatment of choice (Figure 4.22).

Mention must be made of anterior screw fixation of the odontoid. While in the best hands the results may be impressive, the technique requires considerable expertise and sophisticated radiographic control, and undoubtedly has a high rate of complications including a significant mortality (Aebi, Etter and Koscia, 1989). It is even more difficult technically in the case of a pseudarthrosis, where the bone is soft, and type III fractures where a buttress plate may be necessary also. This operation appears to be a relatively malignant treatment of a relatively benign condition.

A vi Traumatic spondylolisthesis of the axis

The anatomical features and historical aspects of this injury were reviewed by Schneider *et al.* in 1965. They referred to Wood Jones's interest in the subject of judicial hanging when he suggested the title, 'ideal' hangman's fracture. Cornish (1968) reported 14 cases, observing that vertical compression and extension forces were involved. He noted the paradox of a 'flexion' injury at a lower level and considered skull traction illogical in the treatment of this injury. This remains true today.

Williams (1975) recognized two types of traumatic spondylolisthesis. The common type is caused by extension and compression and results from falls onto the face or vertex while the body continues to topple. The same effect is produced when the unrestrained car occupant is projected forwards, striking their head against the inside of the vehicle. In this type injury to the spinal cord is uncommon. The true hangman's fracture is caused by extension and distraction and was seen classically when the knot was placed correctly in the submental rather than the subaural position. The modern counterpart is the loose diagonal safety harness (Saldeen, 1967; Taylor, Nade

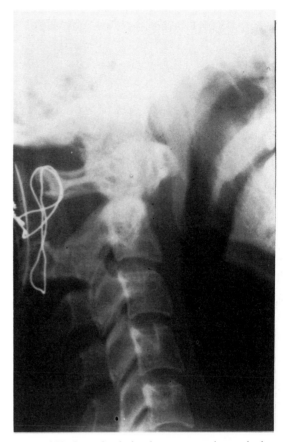

Figure 4.22. Posterior fusion for symptomatic ununited odontoid fracture in a young adult.

and Bannister, 1976). We have seen the distraction type produced by a heavy metal necklace catching in a door handle, and in a motorcyclist who was caught under the jaw by a rope suspended above the roadway (Figure 4.23). (This latter mechanism using a steel wire was often used to detach a dispatch rider from his motorcycle by various resistance groups.) This injury is often associated with cord damage, most commonly a Brown-Sequard syndrome.

Both types of fracture usually heal within 3 months. For undisplaced fractures a rigid orthosis is sufficient. Displaced fractures may be realigned to an acceptable position by appropriate positioning of the neck and if skull traction is used, frequent radiographic control and not more than 2.3 kg (5 lb) weight should be employed.

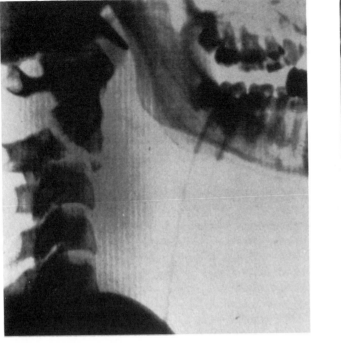

a

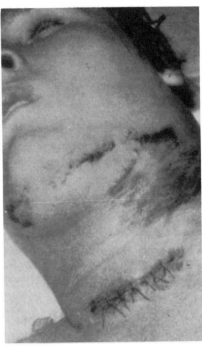

b

Figure 4.23. Hangman's fracture from distraction injury. Note soft tissue injury. (Same patient as Figure 4.12.)

Francis *et al.* (1981) and Effendi *et al.* (1981) have reported large series treated conservatively with few complications and a low incidence of late instability, for which they advocate anterior fusion. In view of the report by White and Moss (1978) of a case undiagnosed for 4 months presenting with anterior subluxation and neurological symptoms on neck flexion, this advice would appear to be appropriate.

A vii Fractures of the body of the axis

As with other vertebral body fractures these heal rapidly with simple supportive treatment.

A viii Subluxation of the axis on the third cervical vertebra

This injury is commonly missed in the adult, and often over-diagnosed in children. The adult injury has no special characteristics, but seems to be overlooked with sufficient frequency to warrant special mention. Any

symptoms usually disappear within a few days and attention is often focused on other injuries. The patient then returns 6 weeks later complaining of pain and clicking in the neck. Surgical fusion at that stage may be the treatment of choice.

'Pseudo-subluxation' between C2 and C3 and to a lesser extent between C3 and C4 is observed frequently in otherwise normal children. Sullivan, Bruwer and Harris (1958) noted a forward glide of 4 mm between the second and third cervical vertebrae in 9 per cent of normal children. Cattell and Filtzer (1965) reported similar findings.

Nevertheless, true subluxation occurs, usually in older children as a result of trauma, as evident by a prevertebral swelling shortly after injury, and later calcification in the interspinous ligament (Figure 4.24). In one of our patients, a boy of 12, neck symptoms were sufficiently severe to justify fusion. At operation the capsules of the facet joints could not be identified and the interspinous ligament was atrophic.

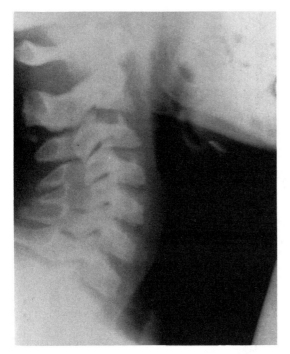

Figure 4.24. Traumatic C2,3 subluxation. Stable after 2 months' conservative treatment. Note calcification in interspinous ligament. (Same patient as Figure 4.10.)

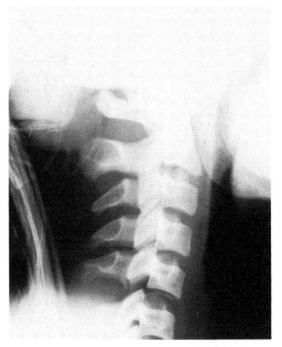

Figure 4.25. Spontaneous reduction by incremental traction. (Same patient as Figure 4.2.)

B Lower cervical spine (C3–T1)

B i Dislocations and fracture dislocations

Skull traction is applied and suitable sedation arranged depending on the patient's age and muscular development. In patients received within a few days of injury traction is begun with 4.5 kg (10 lb) and serial lateral X-rays are taken as weights are increased gradually up to 22.7 or 27.2 kg (50 or 60 lb) (Ducker *et al.*, 1984). The head end of the bed is raised. As the facets commence to distract the supported neck is brought into slight flexion by raising the line of pull. When sufficient distraction has been achieved and confirmed by lateral X-rays, the facets commonly reduce spontaneously (Figure 4.25). Final reduction may be assisted also by a well-timed dose of an intravenous agent such as diazepam or a low dose of propofol, and extension of the neck when the facets have been unlocked by traction.

It is a mistake to extend the neck before there is radiographic confirmation that the facets are sufficiently distracted. As soon as reduction has been achieved the weights are reduced to 2.3 kg (5 lb) and reduction and appropriate extension confirmed on X-ray.

Where there is a unilateral locked facet, altering the line of traction away from the side of the lesion may help. This is one of the advantages of using an outrigger on which the pulley can be moved laterally.

Throughout this procedure the patient's pulse and blood pressure are monitored, repeated neurological examination is carried out, and the patient is asked to report any neurological symptoms. Should the neurological deficit increase, the traction is reduced and manipulation under anaesthesia or open reduction may be carried out. If possible, the latter course is better avoided as an emergency in patients with cord injury as it is associated with increased neurological deficit and mortality (Osti, Fraser and Griffith, 1989). If reduction has not been achieved in three hours (and it is more difficult to achieve in unifacet dislocations where the 'intact' joint may prevent sufficient distraction), we favour manipulation under anaesthetic. Absolute cooperation between the surgeon and the anaethetist is required in this procedure as the timing of full muscle relaxation is essential.

Bilateral dislocations generally are easier to reduce than unilateral locked facets. In the latter case lateral flexion followed by rotation away from the side of the lesion while maintaining long axis traction is an essential part of the procedure. This is followed by rotation of the head towards the side of dislocation and, at the same time, extension. Reduction is often accompanied by an audible click (Evans, 1961).

Kleyn (1984) reported manipulation under anaesthesia in 101 patients, 45 intact or incomplete and 47 with unilateral dislocation, with success in 82 and no complications or neurological loss. While Evans (1983) felt C7, T1 dislocations were difficult if not impossible to reduce in this way, McCoy *et al.* (1984) reported a successful case with almost complete neurological recovery. Men with short, well-muscled necks present the most difficulty in reduction, and McSweeney (personal communication) would not attempt manipulation below C6, particularly in individuals of that type.

Where the injury is more than 48 hours old, reduction on traction may be attempted, but if this is unsuccessful open reduction may be preferable to manipulation (although Evans and McSweeney draw the line at 5 days, personal communication). Neurological deterioration (fortunately temporary) has been reported after open reduction of a unilateral dislocation, and was associated with a large anterior disc fragment, later removed (Venter, 1990).

Unifacet dislocations received some days late may be left unreduced. Mayer (1988) reports good results from this, although Rorabeck *et al.* (1987) do not agree. Our experience is akin to that of Mayer. Certainly it may be safer and better to leave unreduced all dislocations received more than 2 or 3 weeks post injury.

Once reduction has been achieved (or even if it has not) the choice must be made between conservative management and surgical fusion. We favour early posterior fusion for those patients with complete disruption of the posterior ligament complex (including the hidden

flexion injury) and no, or minor, neurological deficit. With conservative treatment, such injuries normally fuse with a kyphotic deformity which, while unattractive to the eye of the clinician, is still safe and symptom free from the point of view of the patient (see Figure 4.13a,b).

Patients with sufficient neurological deficit to require some weeks of inpatient care, and those with complete tetraplegia are treated conservatively, as are those with significant bone injury likely to result in spontaneous fusion, or who are poor anaesthetic risks.

In our hands conservative treatment consists of 4–6 weeks skull traction followed by mobilization in an orthosis–supporting for complete lesions, rigid (e.g. Minerva plaster) for those who will be ambulant and have normal skin sensation and chest function. Flexion extension films may be taken at 6 weeks to assess progress, but in general, once we have embarked on a programme of conservative management, we do not assess stability or change course until 3 months or more from injury. If there is persisting abnormal motion at the level of injury after that length of time we advise posterior fusion.

B ii Vertebral body fractures

Severe burst fractures are commonly associated with significant cord injury and are treated in recumbency with the spine aligned posturally and by light skull traction. As with hyperextension injuries, so with burst fractures, there are those who advocate anterior decompression in some cases (Bohlman and Boada, 1983), and again, sound clinical evidence of the value of this procedure is awaited. With conservative treatment the potential for the recovery of incomplete lesions is unpredictable and unlimited, while Stauffer (1984) has shown that 90 per cent of complete lesions recover at least one level spontaneously, 66 per cent to a full functional grade, without decompression.

Less severe vertebral body fractures together with lateral mass fractures and minor unilateral fracture subluxations may be treated, in the absence of cord injury, by early mobilization in a rigid orthosis. However, the last group particularly are often associated with a good deal of pain and a nerve root lesion, cannot be maintained fully reduced in

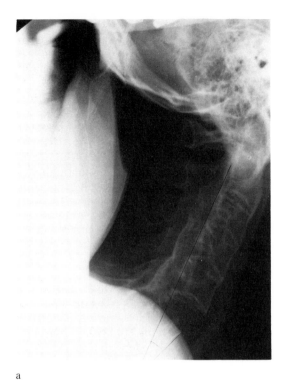

a

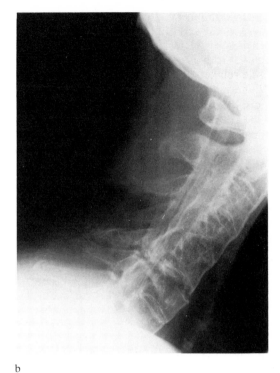

b

c

Figure 4.26. (a) C5,6 fracture. Ankylosing spondylitis. Severe tetraparesis. (b) Postural reduction. (c) Spontaneous healing. Conservative treatment. Little neurological recovery.

an orthosis, and may be managed best by 3 or 4 weeks skull traction in recumbency.

B iii Hyperextension injuries

For those cases with no significant bone injury or displacement potential, the treatment is that of the cord injury and a soft collar is all that is required for the neck. Traction is not indicated unless the spinal column is unstable, in which case it should be in neutral or slight flexion and monitored carefully by serial radiographs.

While there are those (Cloward, 1961) who advocate anterior decompression and/or fusion for hyperextension injuries with neural deficit, there is no statistically significant clinical evidence that such operative treatment aids neurological recovery, nor would consideration of spinal cord pathology lead one to expect it.

B iv Miscellaneous

The British experience of compound injuries of the cervical spine fortunately remains very limited. The topic has been covered in the classic reviews of Lipschitz (1976, stab wounds) and Yashon (1976, missile injuries).

Of fractures of pathological spines, those occurring in association with ankylosing spondylitis are particularly lethal. Among the many problems, gastrointestinal haemorrhage is a frequent complication. Conservative treatment gives best results either by traction in recumbency or halo vest, both requiring extremely careful positioning and radiological and neurological monitoring (Figures 4.26a,b and c).

It has been shown also that the best results are obtained when the patient is cared for in a Spinal Injury Unit (Foo, Sarkarati and Marcelino, 1985; Harding *et al.*, 1985; Broom and Raycroft, 1988; Graham and Van Peteghem, 1989).

Conclusion

One would not wish to give the impression that there is one simple or correct answer to the problems of cervical spine injury. Cervical dislocations in particular are dangerous and sometimes lethal injuries and the behaviour of the cord may be quite unpredictable. While all

forms of management, including no active treatment, give good results in many cases, all are associated on occasion with neurological loss, major or minor, temporary or permanent, complete or incomplete.

We have seen a patient with no significant cord injury develop sudden and complete tetraplegia at the completion of uneventful reduction of a bilateral dislocation by incremental traction 5 days after injury, the neurological loss occurring after reduction had been achieved and the weights had been reduced to 6.4 kg (14 lb). Fortunately, complete recovery occurred within 24 hours. So long as the management is competent, disasters will be few. The cardinal principles are to make the correct diagnosis, and if in doubt, to seek advice from experienced quarters.

Sadly, it remains true, that failure to diagnose and institute appropriate first line management for cervical injuries remains a much greater cause of morbidity and mortality than is failure to intervene with a scalpel.

References

Acikgoz, B., Ozgen, T. and Erbengi, A. (1990) Wrestling causing paraplegia. *Paraplegia*, **28**, 265–268.

Ackroyd, C.E. and Hobbs, C.A. (1979) The use and effectiveness of seat belts. *Journal of Bone and Joint Surgery*, **61B**, 518 (Proceedings).

Aebi, M., Etter, C and Koscia, M. (1989) Fractures of the odontoid process. Treatment with anterior screw fixation. *Spine*, **14**, 1065–1070.

Allen, J.P. (1976) Spinal cord injury at birth. In *Handbook of Clinical Neurology*, 25; (P.J. Vinken and G.W. Bruyn eds.) Amsterdam: North Holland Publishing Co. pp. 155–173.

Anderson, L.D. and D'Alonzo, R.T. (1974) Fractures of the odontoid process of the axis. *Journal of Bone and Joint Surgery*, **56A**, 1663–1674.

Apple, D.F., McDonald, A.P. and Smith, R.A. (1987) Identification of herniated nucleus pulposus in spinal cord injury patients. *Paraplegia*, **25**, 63 (Proceedings).

Arnold, J.G. (1955) Spondylochondrosis of the cervical spine. *Annals of Surgery*, **141**, 872–883.

Askenasy, H.M., Braham, J. and Kosary, I.Z. (1960) Delayed spinal myelopathy following atlanto-axial fracture dislocation. *Journal of Neurosurgery*, **17**, 1100–1104.

Barnes, R. (1948) Paraplegia in cervical injuries. *Journal of Bone and Joint Surgery*, **30B**, 234–244.

Bauze, R.J. and Ardran, G.M. (1978) Experimental production of forward dislocation in the human cervical spine. *Journal of Bone and Joint Surgery*, **60B**, 239–245.

Beatson, T.R. (1963) Fractures and dislocations of the cervical spine. *Journal of Bone and Joint Surgery*, **45B**, 21–35.

Bedbrook, G.M. (1981) *The Care and Management of Spinal Cord Injuries.* Springer Verlag, New York.

Bell, H.S. (1976) Cruciate paralysis. In *Handbook of Clinical Neurology*, **25**, (P.J. Vinken and G.W. Bruyn eds). Amsterdam; North Holland Publishing Co. pp. 391–392.

Bentley, G. and McSweeney, T. (1968) Multiple spinal injuries. *British Journal of Surgery*, **55**, 565–570.

Birney, T.J. and Hanley, E.N. (1989) Traumatic cervical spine injuries in childhood and adolescence. *Spine*, **14**, 1277–1282.

Bohlman, H.H. and Boada, E. (1983) Fractures and dislocations of the lower cervical spine. In *The Cervical Spine*, Philadelphia, J.B. Lippincott Company, pp 232–267.

Bonney, G. (1959) Prognosis in traction lesions of the brachial plexus. *Journal of Bone and Joint Surgery*, **41B**, 4–35.

Bosch, A., Stauffer, E.S. and Nickel, V.L. (1971) Incomplete traumatic quadriplegia. A ten year review. *Journal of the American Medical Association*, **216**, 473–487.

Braakman, R. and Penning, L. (1971) Injuries of the cervical spine. *Excerpta Medica*, 77–97.

Braakman, R. and Penning, L. (1976) Injuries of the cervical spine. In *Handbook of Clinical Neurology*, **25**, (P.J. Vinken and G.W. Bruyn eds). Amsterdam; North Holland Publishing Co. pp. 253–259.

Bracken, M.B., Shepard, M.J., Collins, W.F. *et al.* (1990) A randomised controlled trial of Methylprednisolone or Naxolone in the treatment of acute spinal cord injury. *New England Journal of Medicine,* **322**, 1403–1411.

Brav, E.A. (1936) Voluntary dislocation of the neck. Unilateral rotatory subluxation of the atlas. *American Journal of Surgery*, **32**, 144–149.

Breig, A. (1978) *Adverse Tension in the Central Nervous System.* Stockholm; Almquist and Wiksell; New York; John Wiley and Sons Inc.

Broom, M.J. and Raycroft, J.F. (1988) Complications of fractures of the cervical spine in ankylosing spondylitis. *Spine*, **13**, 763–766.

Burke, D.C. (1971) Hyperextension injuries of the spine. *Journal of Bone and Joint Surgery*, **53B**, 3–12.

Cattell, H.S. and Filtzer, D.L. (1965) Pseudosubluxation and other normal variations in the cervical spine in children. *Journal of Bone and Joint Surgery*, **47A**, 1295–1309.

Chacko, V., Joseph B., Mohanty, S.P. *et al.* (1986) Management of spinal cord injury in a general hospital in rural India. *Paraplegia*, **24**, 330–335.

Cheshire, D. (1969) The stability of the cervical spine following the conservative treatment of fractures and fracture dislocations. *Paraplegia*, **7**, 193–203.

Clark, C.R. and White, A.A. (1985) Fractures of the dens. *Journal of Bone and Joint Surgery*, **67A**, 1340–1348.

Clark, C.R., Igram, C.M., Elkhoury, G.Y. *et al.* (1988) Radiological evaluation of cervical spine injuries. Presented at II Common Meeting of the European and American Sections Cervical Spine Research Society, Marseilles. June 12th–15th 1988.

Cloward, R.B. (1961) Treatment of acute fractures and fracture-dislocations of the cervical spine by vertebral body fusion. A report of eleven cases. *Journal of Neurosurgery*, **18**, 201–209.

Collins, W.F. (1983) A review and update of experimental and clinical studies of spinal cord injury. *Paraplegia*, **21**, 204–219.

Corner, L.M. (1907) Rotary dislocation of the atlas. *Annals of Surgery*, **45**, 9–26.

Cornish, B.L. (1968) Traumatic spondylolisthesis of the axis. *Journal of Bone and Joint Surgery*, **50B**, 31–43.

Crutchfield, W.G. (1938) Treatment of injuries of the cervical spine. *Journal of Bone and Joint Surgery*, **20**, 696–704.

Dall, D.M. (1972) Injuries of the cervical spine. I. Does the type of bony injury affect spinal cord recovery? II. Does anatomical reduction of the bony injuries improve the prognosis for spinal cord recovery? *South African Medical Journal*, **40**, 1048–1056; and **46**, 1083–1090.

Davis, D., Bohlman, H., Walker, A.E. *et al.* (1973) The pathological findings in fatal cranio-spinal injuries. *Journal of Neurosurgery*, **34**, 603–613.

Ducker, T.B. (1976) Experimental injury of the spinal cord. In *Handbook of Clinical Neurology*, **25**, (P.J. Vinken and G.W. Bruyn eds). Amsterdam; North Holland Publishing Co. pp. 9–26.

Ducker, T.B., Belegarrigue, R., Calcman, M. *et al.* (1984) Timing of operative care in cervical spinal cord injury. *Spine*, **9**, 525–531.

Duke, R.F.N., Spreadbury, T.H. (1981) Closed manipulation leading to immediate recovery from cervical spine dislocation with paraplegia. *Lancet*, **2**, 577–578.

Effendi, B., Roy, D., Cornish, B. *et al.* (1981) Fractures of the ring of the axis. A classification based on the analysis of 131 cases. *Journal of Bone and Joint Surgery*, **63B**, 318–327.

Eismont, F.J. and Bohlman, H.H. (1978) Posterior atlanto-occipital dislocation with fractures of the atlas and odontoid process. *Journal of Bone and Joint Surgery*, **60A**, 397–399.

Elliot, G.R. and Sachs, E. (1912) Observation on fracture of odontoid process of axis with intermittent pressure paralysis. *Annals of Surgery*, **56**, 876–882.

Elliott, H.C. (1945) Cross sectional diameters and areas of the human spinal cord. *Anatomical Record*, **93**, 287–293.

Ersmark, H., Dalen, N., Kalen, R. (1990) Cervical spine injuries; A follow-up of 332 patients. *Paraplegia*, **28**, 25–40.

Evans, D.K. (1961) Reduction of cervical dislocations. *Journal of Bone and Joint Surgery*, **43B**, 552–555.

Evans, D.K. (1976) Anterior cervical subluxation. *Journal of Bone and Joint Surgery*, **58B**, 318–321.

Evans, D.K. (1983) Dislocations at the cervico-thoracic junction. *Journal of Bone and Joint Surgery*, **65B**, 124–127.

Evarts, C.M. (1970) Traumatic occipito-atlantal dislocation; report of a case with survival. *Journal of Bone and Joint Surgery*, **52A**, 1653–1660.

Fielding, J.W. (1973) Selected observations on the cervical spine in the child. *Current Practice in Orthopaedic Surgery*, **5**, 31–55.

Foo, D., Sarkarati, M. and Marcelino, V. (1985) Cervical spine cord injury complicating ankylosing spondylitis. *Paraplegia*, **23**, 358–363.

Forsyth, H.F. (1964) Extension injuries of the cervical spine.*Journal of Bone and Joint Surgery*, **46A**, 1792–1797.

Francis, W.R., Fielding, J.W., Hawkins, R.J. *et al.* (1981) Traumatic spondylolisthesis of the axis. *Journal of Bone and Joint Surgery*, **63B**, 313–318.

Frankel, H. (1970) Tracheal stenosis following tracheostomy. *Paraplegia*, **8**, 172–174.

Funk, J.F. and Wells, R.E. (1975) Injuries of the cervical spine in football. *Clinical Orthopaedics and Related Research*, **109**, 50–58.

Gabrielson, T.O. and Maxwell, J.A. (1966) Traumatic atlanto-occipital dislocation; with case report of a patient who survived. *American Journal of Roentgenology*, **97**, 624–629.

Gehrig, R. and Michaelis, L.S. (1968) Statistics of acute paraplegia and tetraplegia on a national scale. *Paraplegia*, **6**, 93–95.

Gehweiler, J.A. Jr, Osborne, R.L. Jr, and Becker, R.F. (1980) *The Radiology of Vertebral Trauma*. Saunders, Philadelphia.

Geisler, W.O., Wynne Jones, M. and Jousse, A.T. (1966) Early management of patients with trauma to the spinal cord. In *Proceedings, Third International Congress of Neurological Surgery of the World Federation of Neurosurgical Societies*. Copenhagen. 1965. (A.C. de Vet, W.F. Kennedy and P.J. Vinken eds.) I.C.S. 110. Excerpta Medica. Amsterdam. pp. 331–339.

Graham, B. and Van Peteghem, P.K. (1989) Fracture of the spine in ankylosing spondylitis; diagnosis, treatment and complications. *Spine*, **14**, 803–807.

Greeley, P.W. (1930) Bilateral (ninety degrees) rotatory dislocation of the atlas upon the axis. *Journal of Bone and Joint Surgery*, **12**, 958–962.

Gregg, T.M. (1967) Organization of a spinal injury unit within a rehabilitation centre. *Paraplegia*, **5**, 163–166.

Grundy, D.J., McSweeney, T. and Francis Jones, H.W. (1984) Cranial nerve palsies in cervical injuries. *Spine*, **9**, 338–343.

Guttmann, L. (1973) *Spinal Cord Injuries. Comprehensive Management and Research*. Oxford: Blackwell Scientific Publicationns. pp. 216–268.

Guttmann, L. and Frankel, H. (1966) The value of intermittent catheterization in the early management of traumatic paraplegia and tetraplegia. *Paraplegia*, **4**, 63–84.

Hachen, H.J. (1974) Emergency transportation in the event of acute spinal cord lesionn. *Paraplegia*, **12**, 33–37.

Hadley, L.A. (1944) Roentgenographic studies of the cervical spine. *American Journal of Roentgenology*, **52**, 173–195.

Hadley, L.A. (1949) Constriction of the intervertebral foramen. *Journal of the American Medical Association*, **140**, 473–476.

Haralson, R.H. and Boyd, H.B. (1969) Posterior dislocation of the atlas on the axis without fracture. *Journal of Bone and Joint Surgery*, **51A**, 561–566.

Harding, J.R., McCall, I.W., Park, W.M. *et al.* (1985) Fracture of the cervical spine in ankylosing spondylitis. *British Journal of Radiology*, **58**, 3–7.

Hardy, A.G. and Rossier, A.B. (1975) *Spinal Cord Injuries.* Stuttgart; Georg Thieme.

Harris, J.H., Edeiken-Monroe B. and Kopaniky, D.R. (1986) A practical classification of acute cervical spine injuries. *Orthopedic Clinics of North America*, **17**, 15–30.

Hays, M.B. and Alker, G.J. (1988) Fractures of the atlas vertebrae; the two part burst fracture of Jefferson. *Spine*, **13**, 601–603.

Holdsworth, F.W. (1963) Fractures, dislocations and fracture-dislocations of the spine. *Journal of Bone and Joint Surgery*, **45B**, 6–20.

Holdsworth, F.W. (1965) Acute injuries of the cervical spine with cord damage. In *Proceedings of the Third International Congress of Neurological Surgeons*, Copenhagen, (A.C. de Vet, W.F.C. Kennedy and P.J. Vinken eds.) *Excerpta Medica*, **110**, 323–325.

Holdsworth, F.W. (1970) Fractures, dislocations and fracture-dislocations of the spine. *Journal of Bone and Joint Surgery*, **52A**, 1534–1551.

Hughes, J.T. and Brownwell, B. (1963) Spinal cord damage from hyperextension injury in cervical spondylosis. *Lancet*, **i**, 687–690.

Iwegbu, C.G. (1983) Traumatic paraplegia in Zaria, Nigeria; The case for a centre for injuries of the spine. *Paraplegia*, **21**, 81–85.

Jackson, R.H. (1927) Simple uncomplicated rotary dislocation of the atlas. *Surgery, Gynecology and Obstetrics*, **45**, 156–164.

Jefferson, G. (1920) Fractures of the atlas vertebra; Report of four cases and a review of those previously recorded. *British Journal of Surgery*, **20**, 407–422.

Jefferson, G. (1940) Discussion on fractures and dislocations of the cervical spine. *Proceedings of the Royal Society of Medicine*, **33**, 657–660.

Jellinger, K. (1976) Neuropathology of cord injuries. In *Handbook of Clinical Neurology*, **25**, (P.J. Vinken and G.W. Bruyn eds). Amsterdam; North Holland Publishing Co. pp. 43–122.

Khan, E.A. and Yglesias, I. (1935) Progressive atlanto-axial dislocation. *Journal of the American Medical Association*, **105**, 348–352.

Kinoshita, H. and Hirakawa, H. (1989) Pathological studies and pathological principles on the management of extension injuries of the cervical spine. *Paraplegia*, **27**, 172–181.

Kleyn, P.J. (1984) Dislocations of the cervical spine; closed reduction under anaesthesia. *Paraplegia*, **22**, 271–281.

Ladd, A.L. and Scranton, P.E. (1986) Congenital cervical stenosis presenting as transient quadriplegia in athletes. *Journal of Bone and Joint Surgery*, **68A**, 1371–1374.

Landelis, C.D. and Van Peteghem, P.K. (1988) Fractures of the atlas; classification treatment and mobility. *Spine*, **13**, 532–541.

Levine, A.M. and Edwards, C.C. (1986) Treatment of injuries in the C1-C2 complex. *Orthopedic Clinics of North America*, **17**, 31–44.

Lipschitz, R. (1976) Stab wounds of the spinal cord. In *Handbook of Clinical Neurology*, **25**, (P.J. Vinken and G.W. Bruyn eds). Amsterdam; North Holland Publishing Co. pp 197–207.

Livingston, M.C. (1971) Spinal manipulation causing injury. A three year study. *Clinical Orthopaedics*, **81**, 82–86.

Louw, J.A., Mafoyane, N.A., Small, B. *et al.* (1990) Occlusion of the vertebral artery in cervical spine dislocations. *Journal of Bone and Joint Surgery*, **72B**, 678–681.

McCall, I.W., Park, W.M. and McSweeney, T. (1973) The radiological demonstration of acute lower cervical injury. *Clinical Radiology*, **24**, 235–240.

McCoy, G.F., Piggot, J., MacAffee, A.L. *et al.* (1984) Injuries of the cervical spine in schoolboy rugby football. *Journal of Bone and Joint Surgery*, **66B**, 500–503.

McDermott, F. (1978) Control of road trauma epidemic in Australia. *Annals of the Royal College of Surgeons of England*, **60**, 437–450.

McSweeney, T. (1971) Stability of the cervical spine following injury accompanied by grave neurological damage. *Proceedings of the Eighteenth Spinal Cord Injury Conference*, Boston; Veterans Association. pp. 61–65.

Marar, B.C. (1974) The pattern of neurological damage as an aid to the diagnosis of the mechanism in cervical spine injuries. *Journal of Bone and Joint Surgery*, **56A**, 1648–1654.

Masini, M., Neto, N.G.F., Neves, E.G.C. (1990) Experience with spinal cord unit in Brasilia, Brazil. *Paraplegia*, **28**, 17–24.

Mayer, P.J. (1988) The management of unilateral cervical facet dislocation. II *Common Meeting of the European and American Sections, Cervical Spine Research Society*, Marseilles, France.

Michaelis, L.S. (1976) Epidemiology of spinal cord injury. In *Handbook of Clinical Neurology*, **25**, (P.J. Vinken and G.W. Bruyn eds.) Amsterdam; North Holland Publishing Co. pp. 141–143.

Munro, D. (1952) *The Treatment of Injuries to the Nervous System.* Philadelphia; W.B. Saunders. pp. 56–169.

Nachemson, A. (1960) Fractures of the axis. *Acta Orthopaedica Scandinavica*, **29**, 1885–217.

Norrell, H.A. (1971) The role of early vertebral body replacement in the treatment of certain cervical spine fractures. *Proceedings of the Eighteenth Spinal Cord Injury Conference*, 35–39.

Osgood, R.B. and Lund, C.C. (1928) Fractures of the odontoid process. *New England Journal of Medicine*, **198**, 61–72.

Osti, O.L., Fraser, R.D. and Griffiths, E.R. (1989) Reduction and stabilisation of cervical dislocations. *Journal of Bone and Joint Surgery*, **71B**, 275–282.

Page, C.P., Story, J.L., Wissinger, J.P. *et al.* (1973) Traumatic atlanto-occipital dislocation. *Journal of Neurosurgery*, **39**, 394–397.

Pearman, J.W. and England, E.J. (1973) *The Urological Management of the Patient following Spinal Cord Injury.* Springfield, Illinois; Charles C. Thomas. pp. 159–183.

Pedersen, V., Muller, P.G., Biering-Sorensen, F. (1989) Traumatic spinal cord injuries in Greenland 1965–1986. *Paraplegia*, **27**, 345–349.

Pepin, J., Bourne, R., Hawkins, R. (1981) Odontoid fractures of the axis with special reference to the elderly patient. *Proceedings of the Cervical Spine Research Society, Orthopaedic Transactions*, **5**, 119 (Abstr)

Phillips, W.A. and Hensinger, R.N. (1989) The management of rotatory atlanto-axial subluxation in children. *Journal of Bone and Joint Surgery*, **71A**, 664–668.

Pierce, D.S. (1969) Spinal cord injury with anterior decompression, fusion and stabilization and early rehabilitation. *Journal of Bone and Joint Surgery*, **51A**, 1675.

Pierce, D.S. and Nickel, V.H. (1977) *Total Care of Spinal Cord Injuries.* Boston; Little, Brown and Company.

Pitman, M.I., Pitman, C.A. and Greenberg, I.M. (1977) Complete dislocation of the cervical spine without neurological deficit. A case report. *Journal of Bone and Joint Surgery*, **59A**, 134–135.

Pratt-Thomas, H.R. and Berger, K.E. (1947) Cerebellar and spinal injuries after chiropractic manipulation. *Journal of the American Medical Association*, **133**, 600–603.

Pringle, R.G. (1974) Fractures of the odontoid process of the atlas. *Journal of Bone and Joint Surgery*, **56B**, 200–201 (Proceedings).

Ramadier, J.O. and Bombart, M. (1964) Fractures et luxations du rachis cervical sans lesions medullaires. Lesions des 5 dernieres vertebres cervicales. *Revue de Chirurgie Orthopedique*, **50**, 3–34.

Ransohoff, J. (1977) Cervical spinal cord injury, medical and surgical therapy. *Proceedings of the Nineteenth Spinal Cord Injury Conference*, 1–5.

Ravichandran, G. (1978) Traumatic single facet subluxation of the cervical spine. *Archives of Orthopaedic and Traumatic Surgery*, **92**, 221–224.

Roaf, R. (1960) A study of the mechanics of spinal injuries. *Journal of Bone and Joint Surgery*, **42B**, 810–823.

Roaf, R. (1963) Lateral flexion injuries of the cervical spine. *Journal of Bone and Joint Surgery*, **45B**, 36–38.

Roaf, R. (1972) International classification of spinal injuries. *Paraplegia*, **10**, 78–84.

Rogers, W.A. (1957) Fractures and dislocations of the cervical spine. An end result study. *Journal of Bone and Joint Surgery*, **39A**, 341–376.

Rorabeck, C.H., Rock, M.G., Hawkins, R.J. *et al.* (1987) Unilateral facet dislocation of the cervical spine; an analysis of the results of treatment in 26 patients. *Spine*, **12**, 23–27.

Saldeen, T. (1967) Fatal neck injuries caused by use of diagonal safety belts. *Journal of Trauma*, **7**, 856–862.

Schaafsma, S.J. (1970) Plexus injuries. In *Handbook of Clinical Neurology*, **7**, (P.J. Vinken and G.W. Bruyn, eds.) Amsterdam; North Holland Publishing Co. pp. 402–429.

Schmaus, H. (1890) Beitrage zur pathologischen

Anatomie der Auchenmarkserchutterung. *Virchows Archiv Abteilung A, Pathologische Anatomie*, **122**, 470–495.

Schneider, R.C. (1955) The syndrome of acute anterior spinal cord injury. *Journal of Neurosurgery*, **12**, 95–122.

Schneider, R.C. (1966) Serious and fatal neurosurgical football injuries. *Clinical Neurosurgery*, **12**, 226–236.

Schneider, R.C., Cherry, G. and Pantek, H. (1954) The syndrome of acute central cervical spinal cord injury with special reference to the mechanism involved in hyperextension injuries of the cervical spine. *Journal of Neurosurgery*, **11**, 546–577.

Schneider, R.C., Gosh, H.O., Norrell, H. *et al.* (1970) Vascular insufficiency and differential distortion of brain and cord caused by cervico-medullary football injuries. *Journal of Neurosurgery*, **33**, 363–375.

Schneider, R.C. and Kahn, E.A. (1956) Chronic neurological sequelae of acute trauma to the spine and spinal cord. Part 1. The significance of the acute flexion or 'tear drop' fracture dislocation of the cervical spine. *Journal of Bone and Joint Surgery*, **38A**, 985–997.

Schneider, R.C., Livingstone, K.A., Cave, A.J.E. *et al.* (1965) Hangman's fracture of the cervical spine. *Journal of Neurosurgery*, **22**, 141–153.

Schneider, R.C., Reifel, E., Chrisler, H.O. *et al.* (1961) Serious and fatal football injuries involving the head and spinal cord. *Journal of the American Medical Assoction*, **177**, 362–367.

Selecki, B.R. and Williams, H.B.L. (1970) *Injuries to the Cervical Spine and Cord in Man.* Sydney; Australasian Medical Publishing Co., Ltd. pp. 14–19.

Sherk, H.J. and Nicholson, J.T. (1970) Fractures of the atlas. *Journal of Bone and Joint Surgery*, **52A**, 1017–1024.

Silver, J.R. (1987) Spinal injuries as a result of sporting accidents. *Paraplegia*, **25**, 16–17.

Silverman, F.N. and Kattan, K.R. (1975) Trauma and no-trauma of the cervical spine in paediatric patients. In *Trauma and No-Trauma of the Cervical Spine.* (K.R. Kattan, ed). Springfield, Illinois; Charles C. Thomas. pp. 206–239.

Spence, K.F., Decker, S. and Sell, K.W. (1970) Bursting atlantal fracture associated with rupture of the transverse ligament. *Journal of Bone and Joint Surgery*, **52A**, 543–549.

Stauffer, E.S. (1984) Neurologic recovery following injuries to the cervical spinal cord and nerve roots. *Spine*, **9**, 532–534.

Stover, S.L. and Fine, P.R. (1987) The epidemiology and economics of spinal cord injury. *Paraplegia*, **25**, 225–228.

Stringa, G. (1964) Traumatic lesions of the cervical spine. Statistics, mechanism, classification. In *Neuvieme Congres International de Chirurgie Orthopedique et de Traumatologie.* Vienna. September 1963. Brussels; Imprimerie des Sciences. pp. 224–252.

Sullivan, R.C., Bruwer, A.J. and Harris, L. (1958) Upper mobility of the cervical spine in children. A pitfall in the diagnosis of cervical dislocation. *American Journal of Surgery*, **95**, 636–640.

Sunderland, S. (1974) Mechanisms of cervical nerve root avulsions in injuries of the neck and shoulder. *Journal of Neurosurgery*, **41**, 705–714.

Sussman, B.J. (1978) Fracture dislocation of the cervical spine. A critique of current management in the United States. *Paraplegia*, **16**, 15–38.

Taylor, A.R. (1951) The mechanism of injury to the spinal cord in the neck without damage to the vertebral column. *Journal of Bone and Joint Surgery*, **33B**, 543–547.

Taylor, A.R. and Blackwood, W. (1948) Paraplegia in cervical injuries with normal radiographic appearance. *Journal of Bone and Joint Surgery*, **30B**, 245–248.

Taylor, T.K.F., Nade, S. and Bannister, J.H. (1976) Seat belt fractures of the cervical spine. *Journal of Bone and Joint Surgery*, **58B**, 328–331.

Torg, J.S., Pavlov, H., Genuario, S.E. *et al.* (1986) Neurapraxia of the cervical spinal cord with transient quadriplegia. *Journal of Bone and Joint Surgery*, **68A**, 1354–1370.

Toscano, J. (1988) Prevention of neurological deterioration before admission to a Spinal Cord Injury Unit. *Paraplegia*, **26**, 143–150.

Vanezis, P. (1989) *Pathology of Neck Injury.* Butterworths. London.

Venter, P.J. (1990) Unilateral facet joint dislocation. Proceedings. *Journal of Bone and Joint Surgery*, **72B**, 741.

Verbiest, H. (1962) Anterior approach in cases of spinal cord compression by old irreducible displacement or fresh fracture of the cervical spine. Contribution to operative repair of deformed vertebral bodies. *Journal of Neurosurgery*, **19**, 389–399.

Verbiest, H. (1973) Anterolateral operations for fractures and dislocations of the cervical spine due to injuries or previous surgical interventions. *Clinical Neurosurgery*, **20**, 334–367.

Von Torklus, D. and Gehle, W. (1972) The upper cervical spine in infancy and childhood. In *The Upper Cervical Spine.* (Translated by L.S. Michaelis.) Stuttgart; Georg Thieme Verlag: London; Butterworths.

Wadia, N.H. (1967) Myelopathy caused by atlanto-axial dislocation. (A study of 28 cases.) *Brain*, **90**, 449–471.

Walsh, J.J. (1967) Symposium. The cost of life. *Proceedings of the Royal Society of Medicine*, **60**, 1212–1215.

Walsh, J.J. (1968) Further experience with intermittent catheterization. *Paraplegia*, **6**, 74–78.

Wang, D., Wu, X., Shi, G. *et al.* (1990) China's first total care unit for the spinal cord injured. *Paraplegia*, **28**, 318–320.

Wannamaker, G.T. (1954) Spinal cord injuries. A review of the early treatment in 300 consecutive cases during the Korean conflict. *Journal of Neurosurgery*, **11**, 517.

Watson, N. (1983) Road traffic accidents, spinal injuries and seat belts. *Paraplegia*, **21**, 63–64.

Webb, J.K., Broughton, R.B.K., McSweeney, T. *et al.* (1976) Hidden flexion injury of the cervical spine. *Journal of Bone and Joint Surgery*, **58B**, 322–327.

Weisl, H. (1972) Unusual complications of skull calipers. *Journal of Bone and Joint Surgery*, **54B**, 143–145.

White, A.A. and Moss, H.L. (1978) Hangman's fracture with non-union and late cord compression. *Journal of Bone and Joint Surgery*, **60A**, 839–840.

White, A.A. and Panjabi, M.M. (1978) The clinical biomechanics of the occipito-atlanto axial complex. *Orthopedic Clinics of North America*, **9**, 867–878.

White, A.A., Southwick, W.O. and Panjabi, M.M. (1976) Clinical instability in the lower cervical spine. *Spine*, **1**, 16–27.

Whitley, J.E. and Forsyth, H.F. (1960) The classification of cervical spine injuries. *American Journal of Roentgenology*, **83**, 633–644.

Williams, J.P.R. and McKibbin, B. (1979) Cervical spine injuries in Rugby Union football. *British Medical Journal*, **2**, 1747.

Williams, T.G. (1975) Hangman's fracture. *Journal of Bone and Joint Surgery*, **57B**, 82–88.

Windle, W.F. (1955) *Regeneration in the Central Nervous System*. Springfield, Illinois; Charles C. Thomas.

Wolman, L. (1964) The neuropathology of traumatic paraplegia. *Paraplegia*, **1**, 233–251.

Yarkony, G.M., Roth, E.J., Meyer, P.R. *et al.* (1990) Spinal cord injury care system: fifteen year experience at the Rehabilitation Institute of Chicago. *Paraplegia*, **28**, 321–329.

Yashon, D. (1976) Missile injuries of the spinal cord. In *Handbook of Clinical Neurology*, **25**, (P.J. Vinken and G.W. Bruyn eds). Amsterdam; North Holland Publishing Co. pp. 209–220.

Yeo, J.D. (1976) A review of experimental research in spinal cord injury. *Paraplegia*, **14**, 1–11.

Yeo, J.D., Payne, W. and Hinwood, B. (1975) The experimental contusion injury of the spinal cord in sheep. *Paraplegia*, **12**, 275–295.

Yeo, J.D., Stabback, S., Mackenzie, B. (1977) Experimental spinal cord injury. *Proceedings of the 6th International Congress on Hyperbaric Medicine*, Aberdeen University, pp 223–232.

Young, J.S. (1978) Initial hospitalization and rehabilitation costs of spinal cord injury. *Orthopedic Clinics of North America*, **9**, 263–270.

5 Cervical orthoses

Robert G. Pringle

Which orthosis – the customer's choice

Continuous skull traction in recumbency remains the most effective and reliable method of immobilizing and controlling the injured cervical spine, not only in conservative management but also as an important part of the pre- and intraoperative regimen of those patients treated surgically. However, in patients who are neurologically intact or who have suffered minimal neurological deficit, early mobilization in an orthosis may be appropriate conservative treatment. In such a case the choice of orthosis is important and not infrequently somewhat arbitrary.

There exists a wide range of orthoses of varying efficacy and reliability, extending from the Sorbo collar through a spectrum of increasing size, rigidity, and clumsiness, to the halo vest and Minerva cast. All share one common failing – they all permit significant movement to occur at all levels, injured and uninjured, of the cervical spine. In addition, most (including even the halo vest in our experience) are capable of being removed or dismantled by the patient, which may be an undesirable feature, particularly with less reliable subjects. In their treatment of cervical spine injuries, clinicians at times appear to be unaware of these problems with unfortunate consequences.

Comparative studies of the effectiveness of soft and Philadelphia collars, Somi, four poster and rigid cervicothoracic braces, and the halo vest (but not including the Minerva jacket) were reviewed by Wolf and Johnson (1983). The studies revealed that no orthosis affords complete immobilization of the neck. The soft collar is of course largely ornamental and provides symptomatic benefit but little real support, while the Philadelphia and Somi devices, both in common use in the UK, permit almost 30 per cent of normal flexion/extension, 66 per cent of tilt, and 45 and 33 per cent of rotation respectively, and cannot be relied upon to control the unstable spine. The four poster and cervicothoracic braces limit flexion/extension to 20 and 12 per cent while still permitting 50 per cent tilt and 20 per cent or more rotation respectively. In these studies the halo vest proved to be much the most effective, and Wolf and Johnson recommended this or the cervicothoracic brace as the treatment of choice for most unstable neck injuries from C1 to T1. Not all would agree with this advice.

Johnson *et al.* (1981) described the cervicothoracic brace as 'uncomfortable to wear, particularly for long term use'. Furthermore, recent studies have shown the Minerva jacket to be at least as effective as the halo vest below C2 and to be less prone to complications (Pringle, El Masri and McClelland, 1988; Benzel, Hadden and Saulsbery, 1989).

What is indisputable is that, while with increasing rigidity of orthosis increasing restriction of flexion/extension in the lower cervical spine may be achieved, complete immobilization is not possible, and translation, subluxation, and recurrent dislocation may take place even in the halo vest. Immobilization of the upper cervical spine by these devices is even less effective. The clinician who relies on any orthosis for treatment of the unstable spine without frequent clinical and radiological monitoring will have cause to regret it.

The halo vest

The first published report of the halo vest came from California (Perry and Nickel, 1959) and referred to its use in treatment of spinal paralysis, while James (1960) from Edinburgh was the first to describe its application to cervical injuries. Since that time there have been numerous reports of its benefits and complications. Koch and Nickel (1978) published the results of a detailed evaluation of motion and forces across the neck in a study of six patients in halo vests and one in a halo cast. Using flexion/extension lateral radiographs, motion in that plane was evaluated in supine and upright positions and averaged 31 per cent of normal at the levels tested (C2 to T1). The greatest individual motion was at C4/5 (7.2°), while there was a gradual symmetrical decrease in motion at the levels proximal and distal to it. The percentage of normal motion was greatest at C2/3 (42 per cent) and least at C7/T1 (20 per cent).

In addition, movement from a position of relative extension to one of relative flexion occurred as the subject transferred from the erect to the supine position. They reported also dramatic changes in the compression–distraction forces across the neck in different positions. These varied from 2.3 kg (5 lb) compression to 7.7 kg (17 lb) distraction in different individuals in the sitting position and averaged 8.4 kg (18.6 lb) variation with change in position. The compression force changed by 1.8–2.7 kg (4–6 lb) with each step in the ambulatory patients.

Wang *et al.* (1988), in a study of 20 normal subjects, found a little more motion at each level than did Koch and Nickel, and in addition were able to study the C1 and C2 levels where flexion/extension range averaged 7.0° and 13° respectively.

With such motion permitted and such forces existing in the orthosis, it is not surprising that redisplacement of fractures and subluxations are not uncommon in the halo vest. This has

been not only the Oswestry experience, but has been reported by others (Whitehill, Richman and Glaser, 1986).

Other complications of the halo vest are not infrequent. Garfin *et al.* (1986) in a series of 179 patients found pin loosening in 36 per cent, pin site infection (20 per cent), pressure sores (11 per cent), nerve injury (2 per cent), dural penetration (1 per cent), dysphagia (2 per cent), cosmetically disfiguring scars (9 per cent), and severe pin discomfort in 18 per cent.

The halo vest is, therefore, not a trouble free, fool-proof, or completely effective way of immobilizing the injured cervical spine. Is the Minerva cast a better alternative?

Minerva and her plaster

Plaster casts of the Minerva type have been the stock in trade of the ambulant management of cervical spine disorders since the beginning of this century, and were described

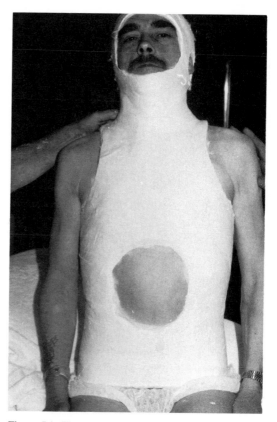

Figure 5.1. The modern Minerva plaster.

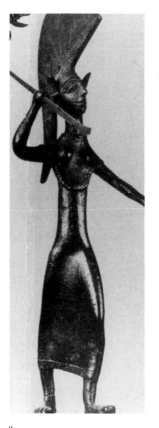 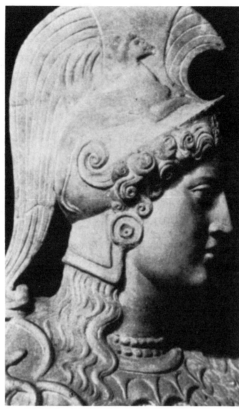

a   b

Figure 5.2 (a) The Etruscan Minerva (New Larousse). (b) The Roman Minerva (Schmidt).

in the treatment of fractures in the works of Bohler (1935), Watson Jones (1940) and Crawford Adams (1960) – although only Crawford Adams used the term 'Minerva'.

Both the Minerva's antecedents and qualifications for the role of fracture treatment are unclear. Why is the plaster so named? At first glance there would seem to be little resemblance between the plaster (Figure 5.1) and Minerva's armour, characterized always by a large crested helmet and only later by a breast plate bearing the head of Medusa given to her by Perseus to fix to the middle of her aegis or shield.

Minerva was a Roman Goddess of Etruscan origin (Figure 5.2a,b), Goddess of the thunderbolt. She became one of the Roman capitoline trinity with Juno and Jupiter, Goddess of elevated thought, literature, art and music, wisdom and intelligence. She soon became identified with the Greek Athene, (Figure 5.3) Goddess of War, Protectress of Heroes and Estate, Goddess of Agriculture, Potters, Weavers, Families, Household, and Health. In

Roman legend, Minerva was born from the head of Jupiter her father, although no mention is made of her mother.

The Greek legend goes into more detail. Zeus having pursued and impregnated Metis the Titaness with Athene, then swallowed Metis whole as he had been warned that if she gave birth to a second child, a son, that child would dethrone him. Later, while walking by Lake Triton, he was seized by a splitting headache. Hermes diagnosed the problem and summoned Hephaestus the Smith, who made a breach in the skull of Zeus with a wedge and beetle. From this breach sprang Athene, fully armed, with a mighty shout (Schmidt, 1980; Bulfinch, 1984; Graves, 1981).

To trace the link between Minerva and her plaster we must go back to 1764 when Levacher, designer of an 18th century standing machine, using slings, traction, cords and windlass for correcting scoliosis, published his description of this device for suspended traction for spinal deformities (Bick, 1968). It

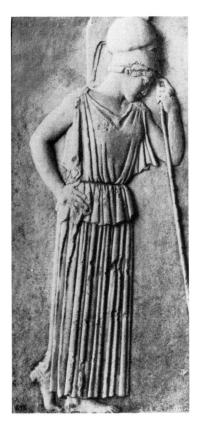

Figure 5.3. Athene (Schmidt).

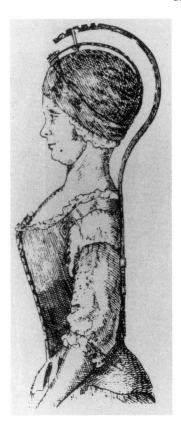

Figure 5.4. Spinal brace with Jury Mast. Levacher 1764 (Bick).

was later named the Jury mast (Figure 5.4). It appears probable that the effect of the Jury mast in giving the appearance of a crest may have led to the appellation 'Minerva', as 100 years later Charriere, the French instrument maker, described a similar orthosis by that name (Figure 5.5).

These early devices were for the correction of spinal deformities. By the 19th century however they were also employed in the treatment of tuberculosis as in the device of Treves (Figure 5.6) – made of felt with a metal back splint and brow strap – and a later illustration in 1914 in *Fraser's Tuberculosis of Bone and Joint* of the Taylor Brace and Jury mast (Figure 5.7). The transition from felt and metal to plaster of Paris may be attributable to Doctor Frederic Calot at Berck-Sur-Mer, who wrote in 1905, 'when surgeons know how to apply an effective plaster of Paris support to the vertebral column, the problem of the treatment of Pott's disease will be solved' (Gauvain, 1913).

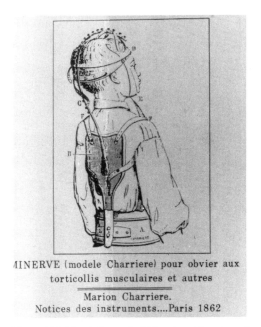

MINERVE (modele Charriere) pour obvier aux torticollis musculaires et autres

Marion Charriere.
Notices des instruments....Paris 1862

Figure 5.5. The 'Minerve' of Charriere (Courtesy of Royal College of Surgeons Library).

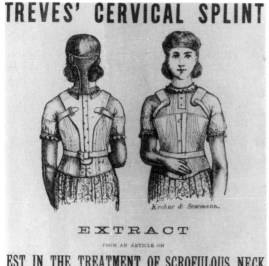

Figure 5.6. Treves' cervical splint (From Krohne and Seseman's Instrument Catalogue 1879, Royal College of Surgeons Library).

Harry Platt (1950) described Frederic Calot (Figure 5.8) as 'a redoubtable and colourful personality who had established his own independent clinic which became known far and wide as the result of his writings and more especially the attractive illustrations in his popular monograph *Orthopaedie Indispensable*, published in 1909 and which went into nine editions'. Calot was an exponent of the injection of cold abscesses with iodiform oil. He wrote enthusiastically about the results in his own hands of the manipulative reduction of congenital hip dislocations and in this field regarded himself as a rival of the great Adolf Lorenz.

Platt called Calot 'the type of virtuoso to be found at every period in all branches of surgery – the man who founds no school and leaves behind no pupils; but his influence on the practice of orthopaedics cannot be discounted'. In Calot's book (Calot, 1910) he is described as Head Surgeon at the Hospital Rothschild, Hospital Cazin, Hospital de l'Oise et des Départements, Dispensaire at the Institut Orthopaedique of Berck.

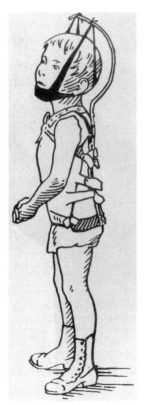

Figure 5.7. Taylor brace and jury mast. (Fraser 1914.)

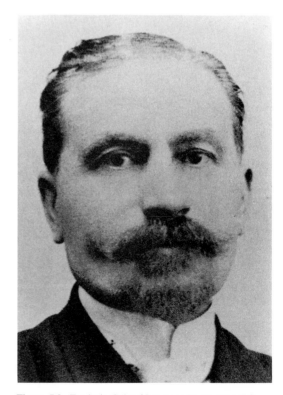

Figure 5.8. Frederic Calot (Courtesy Dr D. Chopin).

His plaster technique was described by Gauvain in 1913 as equalled by few, and it was Calot who favoured the French or Minerva plaster.

The Minerva plaster as used and described by Calot in 1910, (Figure 5.9a and b) was a body jacket moulded to occiput, mastoid and lower jaw; which he described as a funnel enclosing the base of the skull. It was so described by Gauvain in 1913, by Jones and Lovett (1923) and is illustrated by Bohler in 1935.

It is time to cross the Channel. Henry Gauvain (Figure 5.10a and b) was born in Alderney and was appointed as First Superintendent of the new Lord Mayor Treloar's Hospital in 1908 at the age of 30. He had visited Berck, had met Calot, and in 1910 wrote a combined paper with Calve on the management of tuberculosis. He was responsible for introducing splints of Celluloid impregnated muslin which proved very valuable in the treatment of tuberculosis in children. He described Gauvain's test, which is reflex spasm of the abdominal muscles on passive rotation of the inflamed hip.

In 1913 he wrote a paper in *The Lancet* entitled 'The use of plaster of Paris in the mechanical treatment of tuberculous disease of the spine'. In that he wrote 'It is an unfortunate fact that the value of plaster of Paris is so ill recognized in this country and that the technique of its employment is so ill understood'. He included a detailed account of the technique of application of the French or Minerva plaster. He concluded 'the high jacket (Minerva), the application of which I have described, is commonly used on the Continent. While very efficient there are some objections to its use'. He mentions difficulty in chewing, jaw deformity in young children, and goes on to say 'and in male adults the growth of the beard is an intolerable nuisance. To obviate this drawback I have devised another form of high jacket'. This he called the Fillet 'owing to the fact that the head is maintained immobile by retaining a plaster band in the frontal region'. He emphasized the importance still of moulding under the occiput and mastoid (Figure 5.11a,b and c).

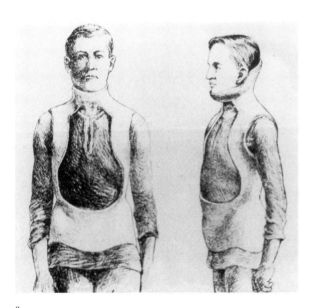

a

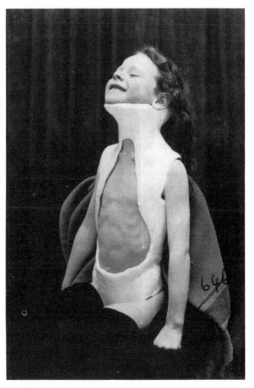

b

Figure 5.9. (a) The Minerva Plaster of Calot (Calot, 1910). (b) The Minerva completed (Gauvain, 1913).

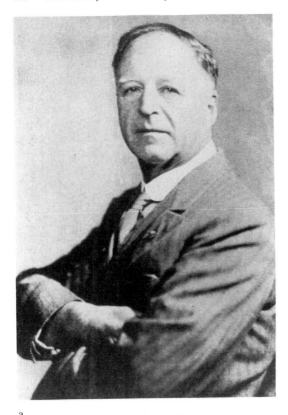
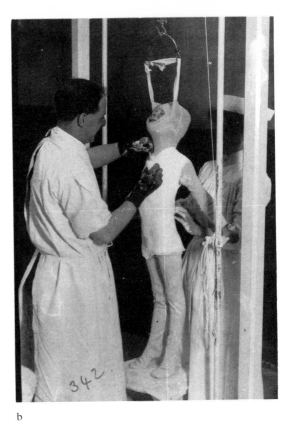

a   b

Figure 5.10. (a) Sir Henry Gauvain (Journal of Bone and Joint Surgery). (b) Henry Gauvain applying a Minerva Plaster (Lord Mayor Treloars Hospital Library).

Thus it would appear that the Minerva plaster, as we now know it is a combination of the Fillet and the French Minerva, was designed for cervical caries, and derives its name from a French orthosis for suspended traction of cervical deformities.

To place this in context Fraser, in 1914, includes also illustrations which reveal that the treatment of cervical caries in other parts of Britain at that time was by plaster of Paris Doll's collar, (Figure 5.12) or alternatively by Thomas' collar (Figure 5.13) and it is interesting to note that the original description of this device is of a collar of soft calf skin stuffed with sawdust, fastened by straps and buckles, and later modified to a collar with a vertical metal strip bent to conform to the chin and chest.

The adoption of the Minerva for the treatment of cervical injury was, therefore, empiric, and its efficiency has only recently been investigated in two studies, one in Louisiana of the Thermo-plastic Minerva brace (Benzel, Hadden and Saulsbery, 1989), and one in Oswestry of the plaster cast (Pringle, El Masri and McClelland, 1988).

The Louisiana study was of 10 patients with spinal injuries (eight operated) who wore halo vests for 6–8 weeks followed by thermoplastic Minerva body jackets (TMBJ). Flexion/extension films were taken prior to removal of the halo jacket and repeated after 2–3 weeks in the TMBJ. At every level except C1/2 (not significant) there was less movement in the TMBJ (average 2.3° against 3.7°). Eight patients preferred the TMBJ for comfort, and there were complaints of pin site loosening infection and scarring, discomfort when attempting to sleep, and neck pain in the halo vest.

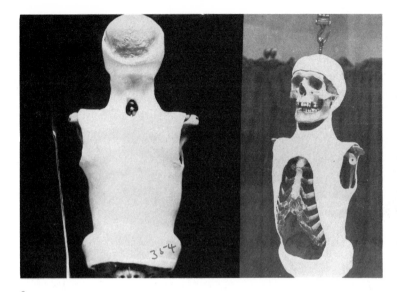

a

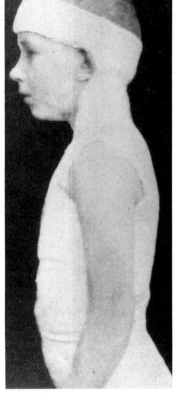

b

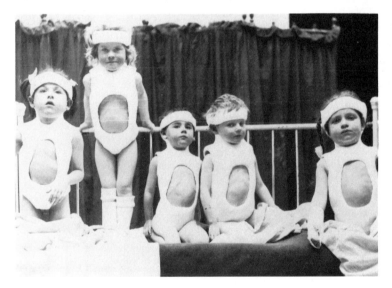

c

Figure 5.11. (a) Gauvain's 'Fillet' plaster (Lord Mayor Treloars Hospital Library). (b) Fillet plaster (Fraser, 1914). (c) Fillet plasters–some of Gauvain's patients (Lord Mayor Treloars Hospital Library).

The Oswestry study included one normal and 15 injured subjects – the latter assessed by lateral X-rays in flexion and extension, in and out of plaster on removal of the cast after 6 weeks in 14 cases and 2 in one (Table 5.1).

The Minerva plaster proved free of complications. In particular, studies of vital capacity were made on several patients in the lying, sitting and standing positions, and no significant impairment of this function was found.

In the normal subject immediately after application of the plaster, no significant motion between C2 and C6 was present in transferring from standing to sitting or supine positions. Three degrees of true flexion were present at the occiput C1 level and similar motion occurred on transfer from standing to supine. At C1/2, 2° and at C6/7, 4° of paradoxical movement, that is to say extension on capital flexion took place. The negative values have been encircled (Table 5.2). The total movement overall was paradoxical and the average segmental movement was –0.5°. This phenomenon of paradoxical motion or snaking

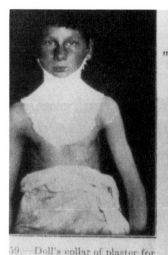

Figure 5.12. The Dolls collar (Fraser, 1914).

"The Doll's Collar" used in th
Shropshire Open Air Hospital
very simple and effective. T
patient is only partially sus
pended and the illustration d
cribes its application. It m
leave the shoulders free play

59.—Doll's collar of plaster for

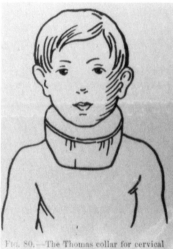

Figure 5.13. Thomas' collar (Fraser, 1914).

of support and fixation may be obtained
by collars. Various materials have been
used for this purpose—poroplaster, etc.
The Thomas collar is the best of this
type of support, and it is the only one
which will be described. The original
Thomas collar was made by stuffing a
tube of soft calf-skin with sawdust, the
diameter being greatest beneath the
chin, and smallest under the ears. It
was secured at the back of the neck
with straps and buckles. A more efficient collar is made by cutting out from
a thin sheet of steel a metal pattern
wide enough to reach from the sternum
to the chin in front, and from the back
of the neck to the occiput. The edges of

FIG. 80.—The Thomas collar for cervical

Table 5.1 Patients in Minerva series

No.	Age (years)	Diagnosis
I	22	C7/T1 Fracture dislocation
II	26	C5/6 Burst fracture
III	19	C5 Burst fracture
IV	48	C6/7 Unifacet fracture dislocation
V	15	C4 Burst fracture
VI	63	C6/7 Unifacet fracture dislocation
VII	15	C5/6 Fracture subluxation (fusion)
VIII	17	C2 Hangman's fracture
IX	49	C2 Lamina fracture
X	69	C2 Dens–lamina fracture
XI	32	C2 Dens fracture
XII	20	C6 Burst fracture
XIII	23	C6/7 Bilateral facet subluxation
XIV	49	C5/6 Unifacet dislocation
XV	41	C5 Burst fracture

Table 5.2 Movement in plaster (in degrees) in a normal subject

Level	Sitting Flexion/extension	Standing	Supine
0–C1	3	0	3.5
C1–C2	-2	0	0
C2–C3	0	1	0
C3–C4	-1	1	0
C4–C5	0.5	0	1
C5–C6	0.5	-2	0
C6–C7	-4	-5	-3
Total	-3	-3	-0.5
Average	-0.5	-0.5	0

Table 5.3 Flexion/extension (in degrees)

| Level | Minerva | Halovest | | |
	Pringle et al. (1988)	Wang et al. (1988)	Koch and Nickel (1978)	Johnson et al. (1981)
0–1	4.0 (mm)	7.0		
1–2	1.3 (mm)	12.8		3.6
2–3	2.1	10.5	4.7	2.2
3–4	3.6	11.1	5.3	2.6
4–5	3.7	11.3	7.2	3.3
5–6	2.2	13.8	5.8	6.5
6–7	2.1	18.6	5.0	2.6

was observed in other subjects in this series and was noted also by Johnson *et al.* (1981) in their study of halo vests.

In the injured patients the average motion at uninjured levels below C2 was similar to that reported for the halo vest by Johnson and less than that reported by Koch and Nickel (1978) and by Wang *et al.* (1988) (Table 5.3) namely between 0.75° (C6/7) and 4° (C4/5), representing between 40 per cent (C2/3) and 5 per cent (C6/7) of the movement occurring at the same levels in the same patient after removal of the casts. No displacement of any injury took place in this series.

Koch and Nickel (1978) in fact compared movement in the orthosis with normal values, whereas the Oswestry studies measured the percentage restriction in and out of plaster. If the movement in plaster in the Oswestry subject is compared with the normal, the Minerva would appear to be significantly superior (Table 5.4).

Once the patient is settled into the plaster it appears to permit an alarming amount of head movement as the patient learns to 'drop' the chin inside the cast. The radiographic studies indicated that free capital flexion of this type was not accompanied by cervical flexion below C1 and may indeed be associated instead with a little paradoxical extension. This movement not only adds to the patient's comfort, but may also mean the patient is less troubled by stiffness on removal of the Minerva than after a period in the halo vest.

This phenomenon of capital flexion may mean also that Gauvain was correct in his design of the Fillet, at least for the control of the neck below C2.

Watson Jones (1940) knew this, and describes cutting the plaster away beneath the chin. It is not necessary to have a firm support

Table 5.4 Flexion/extension (per cent limitation)

| Level | Minerva | | Halovest (Koch) |
	of subject	of normal	
0–1	30		
1–2	63		
2–3	62	82.5	58
3–4	65	80	58
4–5	60	81.5	62
5–6	70	90	72
6–7	65	90	74

under the chin. It is simply necessary to have a brow band and a plaster moulded in such a way as to prevent cervical flexion by holding the head so that capital flexion only is permitted with an axis of rotation at the occiput C1 level.

Bearing this in mind it should be possible to design a modular orthosis whose fitting to an individual patient would require only a well fitting vest and the localization of the axis at the appropriate level under X-ray control. With practice this device might become more sophisticated until it could be tailored to exert appropriately variable control for injuries of different severity at different levels in the neck.

Conclusion

If a neck needs immobilizing, it needs immobilizing properly, and there is in the author's opinion, little place for the intermediate devices of the Somi type which are both relatively ineffective and cumbersome. The halo vest and the Minerva are the treatments of choice in the ambulant management of the unstable cervical spine.

From the available evidence it would appear that the halo vest may be more effective in immobilizing injuries above C2, but that the Minerva is safer, more comfortable, more free of complications, and more reliable for injuries below that level. Both devices however require considerable skill in application and maintenance and the final decision in each case will depend to some extent on the resources available and the patient's preference (Pringle, 1990).

It is not necessary to rely on submental pressure, which is painful and difficult to tolerate, to obtain relatively effective control of cervical flexion. Future orthoses should be designed to avoid such pressure, and to concentrate on localization of the axis of movement and control of the head, in combination with comfort and difficulty in removal of the orthosis by the patient.

References

Benzel, E.C., Hadden, T.A., Saulsbery, C.M. (1989) A comparison of the Minerva and Halo jackets for stabilisation of the cervical spine. *Journal of Neurosurgery*, **70**, 411–414.

Bick, E.M. (1968) *Source Book of Orthopaedics.* New York, Hafner.

Bohler, L. (1935) *The Treatment of Fractures.* John Wright, Bristol.

Bulfinch, T. (1984) *Myths of Greece and Rome.* London, Penguin Books.

Calot, F. (1910) *L'Orthopaedie Indispensable.* Paris, Maloine.

Crawford Adams, J. (1960) *Outline of Fractures Including Joint Injuries.* Edinburgh, E & S Livingstone Ltd.

Fraser, J. (1914) *Tuberculosis of the Bones and Joints in Children.* London, A and C Black.

Garfin, S.R., Botte, M.J., Waters, R.L. *et al.* (1986) Complications in the use of the Halo fixation device. *Journal of Bone and Joint Surgery*, **68A**, 320–325.

Gauvain, H.J. (1913) The use of Plaster of Paris in the mechanical treatment of tuberculosis disease of the spine. *Practitioner*, **90**, 190–202.

Graves, R. (1981) *Greek Myths.* London, Cassell.

James, J.I.P. (1960) Fracture dislocation of the cervical spine. *Journal of the Royal College of Surgeons, Edinburgh*, **5**, 232.

Johnson, R.M., Owen, J.R., Hart, D.L. *et al.* (1981) Cervical orthoses. A guide to their selection and use. *Clinical Orthopaedics*, **154**, 34–45.

Jones, Sir R. and Lovett, R.W. (1923) *Orthopaedic Surgery.* London, Henry Frowde and Hodder and Stoughton.

Koch, R.A. and Nickel, V.L. (1978) The Halo vest: an evaluation of motion and forces across the neck. *Spine*, **3**, 103.

New Larousse, (1970) *Encyclopaedia of Mythology.* London, Paul Hamlyn.

Perry, J., Nickel, V.L. (1959) Total cervical spine fusion for neck paralysis. *Journal of Bone and Joint Surgery*, **41A**, 37–60.

Platt, H. (1950) Orthopaedics in Continental Europe 1900–1950 the changing pattern. *Journal of Bone and Joint Surgery*, **32B**, 573.

Pringle, R.G., El Masri, W.S., McClelland, M.R. (1988) The Minerva plaster and its effect on cervical spine movement. II *Common meeting of the European and American section. Cervical Spine Research Society*, Marseilles June 12–15.

Pringle, R.G. (1990) Review article Halo v Minerva–which orthosis? *Paraplegia*, **28**, 38–42.

Schmidt, J. (1980) *Larousse Greek and Roman Mythology.* New York, McGraw-Hill Book Company.

Wang, G.J., Moskal, J.T., Albert, T. *et al.* (1988) The effect of Halo vest length on stability of the cervical spine. *Journal of Bone and Joint Surgery*, **70A**, 357–360.

Watson Jones, R. (1940) *Fractures and Joint Injuries.* Edinburgh, E and S Livingstone.

Whitehill, R., Richman, J.A., Glaser, J.A. (1986) Failure of immobilisation of the cervical spine by the halo vest. *Journal of Bone and Joint Surgery*, **68A**, 326–332.

Wolf, J.W., Johnson, R.M. (1983) Cervical orthosis. In *The Cervical Spine* (The Cervical Spine Research Society ed.). Philadelphia, J.P. Lippincott & Co. pp. 54–61.

6 Soft tissue injuries

Nature has a constant tendency to repair the injuries to which her structures have been subjected.
                    John Hilton. (Rest and Pain 1864)

Introduction

The supporting ligaments and muscles of the cervical spine can be damaged by injury to a degree short of that necessary to cause fracture or fracture–dislocation of the vertebrae. Patients with such injuries are seen every day in accident units and orthopaedic departments. Lacking the striking neurological signs of cord damage or the radiologically graphic appearances of vertebral displacement, they tend to be treated dismissively; their initial management is often perfunctory and their continuing attendances and complaints greeted with dismay. These attitudes communicate themselves to the patients, who respond with resentment, and a feeling of guilt which exhibits itself as aggression. When, as often happens, the original injury is the source of litigation, the combined resentment of patient and doctor creates a situation in which accurate clinical assessment is impossible and the treatment unrewarding. Much of the blame for this unfortunate state of affairs lies with the use of the term 'whiplash injury' (Crowe, 1928; Gotten, 1956; Zatskin and Kreton, 1960; Knapper, 1964). The term is loose and emotive. Lawyers and laymen love it; so, to their shame do many orthopaedic surgeons. It is used as a convenient shorthand on the grounds that everybody knows what it means. But everybody does not know what it means. It was not coined to describe any soft tissue neck strain sustained in a car accident. Its author later apologized, but by then it was too late. Its use should be regarded as biomechanical illiteracy.

These injuries are caused by acceleration forces, unaccompanied by deceleration beyond that imposed by normal anatomical structures (McNab, 1964). When the head is forcibly flexed the chin strikes the chest before the tension limits of the posterior complex have been reached. If the head is laterally flexed to the shoulder similar considerations apply, reinforced in this direction by the locking mechanism of the apophyseal joints (Veleanu, 1975) (see Chapter 1). Only if external force is applied does the point of contact between chin and chest, or head and shoulder, become the fulcrum around which continuing leverage is applied. If the neck is hyperextended nothing will stop the head until it strikes the upper part of the back. This is usually beyond the normal range of movement, and injuries can result, ranging in severity from soft tissue strain to cord damage with tetraplegia. If extension of the neck is already restricted by spondylosis or ankylosing spondylitis, or if the vertebral arteries are brittle from atherosclerosis, a fracture and a significant cord lesion can follow extension even within the apparently normal range (Taylor and Blackwood, 1948).

Soft tissue injuries can be classified as:

1 Acceleration extension sprains in normal spines.
  Accleration extension sprains in abnormal spines.
2 Acceleration flexion sprains in normal adult spines.

Acceleration flexion sprains in children's spines.

Acceleration flexion sprains in abnormal spines.

3 Lateral flexion injuries with rotation.

Acceleration extension injuries

Pathogenesis

In the middle of the nineteenth century passengers on railway trains began to present a new type of injury. When a stationary train started with a jerk the passenger's head was thrown backwards. When the train ran into another ahead of it the passengers in the leading train suffered similarly. The term 'railway spine' appeared; and the railway companies were inundated with claims for compensation – even the jolting of trains over points was incriminated as a cause of the syndrome. The parallel today is apt. Acceleration extension injuries to the neck are usually low velocity injuries. Hyperextension injuries causing tetraplegia are a different matter and will be considered separately.

The mechanism of injury has been extensively studied (Roaf, 1960; McNab, 1964; 1971; Brain and Wilkinson, 1967; Marar, 1974; Sunderland, 1974; Wickstrom and La Rocca, 1974). Many of these studies have been on experimental animals, some on cadavers. The very nature of the injury precludes findings in patients, except in rare instances (Howcroft and Jenkins, 1977).

The findings may be summarized:

1 Hyperextension injuries alone do not damage the spinal cord (in the normal spine), but may injure the nerve roots.
2 Inward bulging of the ligamentum flavum occurs during normal full extension of the neck, as does inward bulging of the dura. In themselves these corrugations are not significant in acceleration extension injuries (Taylor, 1951; Breig, 1960).
3 The apophyseal joints may be fractured by compression and, in the experimental animal, damage to articular cartilage and sub-chondral bone can be seen (Wickstrom, Rodriguez and Martinez, 1968). It is an uncommon clinical finding.
4 The anterior and posterior longitudinal ligaments are stretched, the anterior more

severely than the posterior. The anterior longitudinal ligament may be torn away from the annulus of the intervertebral disc. There may be haemorrhage beneath the prevertebral fascia.
5 The longus cervicis, longus capitis, scalene and sternomastoid muscles may be torn and swollen by haematoma. The nerve to the rhomboids runs through the scalenus medius and damage to the nerve here may account for the persistent periscapular pain of which many patients complain.
6 The vertebral arteries may be stretched causing temporary ischaemia of the medulla and hind-brain.
7 The sympathetic trunk may be stretched, producing Horner's syndrome.
8 Small bony fragments may be avulsed from the anterior margins of the vertebral bodies, indicating that the anterior longitudinal ligament has been torn away from its bony attachment at that point. In patients this radiographic sign is significant only when there is no other evidence of cervical spondylosis. Annular tearing may predispose to disc degeneration and prolapse, producing later, perhaps discrete, osteophytes.
9 These observations apply to the normal spine. If the acceleration extension injury occurs to a spondylotic spine the limits of elasticity are reached much sooner. The damage is correspondingly more severe.

Clinical features

The characteristic clinical picture of a patient with an acceleration extension injury can now be interpreted in the light of these observations.

The patient is usually a front seat passenger in a car. Seat belts of the inertia type are useful in that they slow the forward shift of the trunk. Rigid seat belts, worn loosely, produce sudden deceleration as violent as contact with the dashboard. The whole question of 'packaging' passengers in motor cars is complex; but it is absurd that fragile glass objects can be packed and despatched in safety while a human being in a car is rattled like a pea in a pod. The driver is less frequently injured because his arms are braced by the steering wheel. A head rest is of protective value only if it projects above the level of the passenger's occiput.

The vehicle is either stationary or moving slowly when it is struck from the rear by another. The leading car and its occupants are accelerated forward but the unsupported head is thrown back. The victim often does not feel immediate pain, indeed he, or she, usually gets out of the car to remonstrate with the driver behind. Examination then will reveal no restriction of neck movement.

Within a period of time varying from a few minutes to two hours or more, neck pain begins. This delay is probably due to the development of traumatic oedema and bleeding in the affected soft tissues. Protective muscle spasm follows and by the time the patient is seen and examined in hospital, neck stiffness is apparent. Other symptoms, usually headache, often radiation of pain into the shoulders, paraesthesis or pain in the arms and hands, pain between the shoulder blades and even low back pain may appear.

Objective physical signs are few. Neck movement, in the early period, is restricted in all directions. With time the restriction is decreased to one or two arcs of movement. Extension is almost always restricted and limited rotation to one or other side is slow to resolve. Neurological signs in this early period are uncommon, but significant when present.

Radiology

X-rays are of value in excluding fractures and fracture dislocations, but there are few pathognomonic appearances of acceleration extension injuries. There may be flattening or even reversal of the normal lordotic curve. Soft tissue swelling in front of the spine may be seen. The distance between the pharynx and the lower margin of the anterior body of C3 shoud not exceed 5 mm (Weir, 1975; Babcock, 1976).

When muscle spasm has subsided, flexion and extension lateral films can be taken. They rarely demonstrate abnormal yawning of the anterior disc space in extension, but in a spondylotic spine may reveal segmental restriction of movement, or hypermobility in segments adjacent to a stiff part of the neck.

Management

When the patient is first seen in hospital, treatment consists of reassurance, splinting and analgesia. The reassurance must be firm but not dismissive. Phrases such as 'You have not broken your neck, but have bruised the supporting ligaments' are comforting. Expressions such as 'There is nothing wrong', when the patient knows there is, are bad; and create, from the beginning, the atmosphere of mutual distrust which too often complicates the long-term management. Such reassurance can only be given after thorough clinical and radiological examination. The presence of other injuries, more apparent at the time, should not interfere with an adequate neurological assessment. The neck will be stiff and painful long after the abrasions and the meticulously sutured lacerations have healed.

The neck must be supported by a collar, fitted in slight flexion or whichever is the most comfortable position. 'Home-made' sorborubber collars or any of the available commercial collars are equally satisfactory. Changes in fashion have made obsolete the method recommended by Watson-Jones in the first edition of his book, when he advised that 'the patient's stiff collar can be opened out and used as a splint' (Watson-Jones, 1940).

If the pain is severe, rest in bed with the neck supported between firm pillows, reinforced with analgesics and muscle relaxants, for a few days may obviate prolonged invalidism. I have no personal experience of the use of systemic or local steroids, chymotrypsin or phenylbutazone as agents to diminish soft tissue swelling in this early phase. The idea is theoretically attractive. Light traction applied via a halter reinforces the splinting affect of pillows or sandbags. Traction of a degree usually carried out for chronic neck pain will aggravate discomfort in the acute phase of extension injury.

It may be argued that such management over-treats an essentially benign condition, may imprint the patient with the idea that his life hangs but by a thread, and may create a chronic over-preoccupation with his health. I do not accept this. In my experience patients who haunt orthopaedic departments with symptoms disproportionate to their physical signs are patients who have been treated perfunctorily from the time of their accident.

Far from reassuring, a dismissive attitude engenders fear and anxiety. A common, and alas, well justified complaint of patients is that the doctor did not tell them anything. The doctor, who is 'too busy' to explain, in simple but not condescending terms, what he or she thinks is the diagnosis and what ought to be the treatment, should not be practising medicine.

After the acute pain has settled many patients will have residual neck pain and stiffness, with or without radiation of pain. Wearing a collar until the symptoms have subsided is sufficient treatment for the majority. When residual stiffness is a problem, physiotherapy in the form of traction, instruction in exercises and deep friction massage is effective.

Prognosis

It has been known for a long time that a substantial number of these patients do badly, with up to 45 per cent experiencing residual symptoms 5 years after injury, and over 2 years after litigation has been resolved (McNab, 1964; Hohl, 1974). These earlier reports were written before seat belts and head restraints became standard equipment in motor cars, and one would have hoped that their introduction reduced the frequency and severity of these injuries. That does not seem to have happened (Greenfield and Illfield, 1977; Deans *et al.*, 1987).

Attempts have been made to identify clinical or radiographic features in the recently injured patient, which can assist in prognosis. Hohl's seminal paper describes pain or numbness radiating into the arms as significant in predicting a long duration of symptoms, but felt that the presence or absence of abnormal physical signs at first examination were not significant. In his series, age was of no consequence but women tended to recover more slowly than men (Hohl, 1974). Greenfield and Illfield (1977) also found that the patient's age had no effect on the final outcome, and that the symptom of pain radiating between the shoulder blades was the only finding consistent with a poor prognosis.

The radiographic signs have been assessed. Greenfield and Illfield found that loss of the normal lordotic curve bore no relation to the

time to recovery, but Hohl wrote that a break in lordosis at one segment was significant. Norris and Watt (1983) assessed 61 cases within 7 days of injury and divided them into three clinical groups; those with symptoms but no signs; those with symptoms and a stiff neck; and those with neurological signs. Of the eight patients in the last group, six were no better or worse after their litigation had been settled. They found a higher incidence of radiographic abnormality in this third group, and felt that alteration of the cervical curve was associated with a poor result. Perhaps more importantly, they found that 40 per cent of the third group showed pre-existing degenerative change on the neck radiographs, against 26 per cent in their first group.

Despite documented evidence that there is little correlation between radiographic degeneration and clinical presentation, lawyers wish to know whether neck injuries will result in the development, or the accelerated development, of degenerative joint or intervertebral disc disease. With age of course these changes become universal, and the incidence accelerates with age. Whereas 6 per cent of people between 30 and 40 years old show radiographic degeneration, this incidence rises to 25 per cent between 40 and 50 years old (Friedenberg and Miller, 1963).

Hohl (1974) found that 39 per cent of his patients developed radiographic changes during his follow-up period of a minimal 5 years after injury. This is more than would be expected from normal ageing, but he did not find correlation between radiographic change and residual symptoms.

Accepting that symptoms can persist for over 5 years in up to 45 per cent of people so injured, it remains to consider what effect litigation itself has on continuing symptoms. McNab was in no doubt that it had no effect (McNab, 1964, 1971, 1973). Other authors have not been so sure (Breck and Van Norman, 1971; Hodge, 1971; Jeffreys, 1991). Norris and Watt (1983) found that all of their third group pursued litigation while only half of their first group did. Breck and Van Norman (1971) found that the duration of treatment in litigants was four times as prolonged as in non-litigants, and Hohl (1974) reported that 83 per cent of those whose claim had been settled within 6 months of the accident were symptom-free at his review against 38 per cent of those whose lawsuits dragged on more than 18 months.

Norris and Watt (1983) felt that those patients injured in a stationary vehicle did worse; and Grundy (Hodgson and Grundy, 1989) has pointed out that the stationary victim of a rear end impact is that rarity in road accidents, totally blameless in the eyes of the law. Grundy's long-term review paints the most pessimistic picture of all, with 10 per cent of patients having to change their occupation or modify their leisure activities because of persistent pain.

Acceleration extension injuries in cervical spondylosis

Many patients with symptoms attributable to cervical spondylosis give a history of injury, but many do not. The development of degenerative changes in patients who have sustained soft tissue injury may be due to normal ageing (Hohl, 1974; 1975). Cervical spondylosis, (and lumbar spondylosis) is seen in patients who earn their living by heavy manual labour (building labourers, coal miners and orthopaedic surgeons) earlier than in those who lead a sedentary life. The clinical syndrome of cervical spondylosis can be precipitated by injury, although asymptomatic radiological changes existed before the injury.

If neck movement is restricted by degenerative changes, strain will fall upon the anterior and posterior longitudinal ligaments before normal full extension is reached. There may be fibrous or bony ankylosis between vertebral bodies, imposing rigidity on the affected segments and greater leverage on those remaining mobile. Such a spine is vulnerable to extension forces which would have no effect on a normal spine.

A patient so afflicted, experiencing an apparently minor extension acceleration injury, will present a very different clinical picture from that seen in a young patient. The onset of pain will be quicker. The pain will be more severe. The radiation of pain into the head, shoulders and arms will be more often seen, as may be objective signs of nerve root damage. Diminution of the biceps or supinator jerk is a common finding reflecting the high incidence of spondylotic changes in the C5/6/7 segments of the spine. Demonstrable muscle

weakness is less often found but a careful search may well reveal diminished sensation in the affected dermatomes (Burke, 1971).

The symptoms of neck pain, stiffness and radiating pain persist for a long time and tend to recur after apparent remission. Restriction of neck movement, initially almost complete, will remain even after pain has subsided (although such restriction of movement could have been present before the accident).

Management of these patients is difficult. The natural history is not one of eventual resolution, but one of remission and relapse over a depressingly long period. Symptomatic relief in the early stages is afforded by a collar but prolonged relief from wearing a collar is unlikely. A common fault is to provide a collar which is too deep, forcing the neck into extension. Most of these patients are comfortable with the neck slightly flexed. The collar does not splint the neck (Johnson *et al.*, 1977, and see Chapter 5).

Other forms of physical treatment, heat, massage, exercises and traction often help and if one method is not successful the others should be tried in turn. This completely pragmatic treatment is justified by experience. Traction must be used with caution, and manipulation with circumspection.

If the sagittal diameter of the cervical spinal canal is shallow, the cord is vulnerable and cervical myelopathy may follow injury. The mean sagittal diameter at C5 is 15 mm (Burrows, 1963), and values less than this imply vulnerability. The diameter may have been further narrowed by the posterior vertebral osteophytes or the thickened ligamentum flavum of spondylosis (Pallis, Jones and Spillane, 1954; Edwards and La Rocca, 1983; Ehni, 1984). One quarter of patients with cervical myelopathy seen at one neurosurgical centre gave a history of injury (Gupta, 1987).

The ultimate cause of the myelopathy is presumably vascular Tokarz and Stachowski, 1974). The vertebral artery, particularly the atheromatous vertebral artery, is at risk in the spondylotic neck. If the maximum strain falls on the segment at which level the feeder branch to the anterior spinal artery leaves the parent trunk, an area of the cord may be infarcted. The level, and number of such feeder vessels is so variable (the radicular branches of the vertebral artery however, which are constant, may be damaged and cause an ischaemic radiculopathy) that it seems that the chances of acquiring an avascular myelopathy are fortuitous. Support for this hypothesis comes from cases of fatal tetraplegia following hyperextension injury to the spondylotic spine where often the only macroscopic lesion is a tell-tale haematoma anterior to the dura at the level of tetraplegia (Scott, 1963).

Damage to the main vertebral trunk is less common. The relative infrequency of spondylotic changes in the upper three cervical segments where the vertebral artery is at its most vulnerable in its sinuous passage from the foramen transversarium of the axis to the foramen in the posterior atlanto-occipital membrane, minimizes the danger. One of my patients developed a lateral medullary syndrome. Another patient showed signs of vertebrobasilar insufficiency immediately after injury, which rapidly subsided after a few days' rest in bed.

Tetraplegia without bony damage

The additional force of a blow on the head causing hyperextension of the spondylotic neck, leading to tetraplegia without fracture of the spine, is now a well recognized and documented phenomenon, since the original paper of Taylor and Blackwood (1948). Taylor (1951) was of the opinion that the infolding of the flavum was the significant mechanism in causing the cord lesion, although Breig (1960) has since demonstrated that much of this apparent infolding is a normal alteration of the outline of the dura in extension of the neck. Other observers have suggested that in addition to yawning open of the spine anteriorly there must be posterior displacement of one vertebra on another before the cord can be injured (Perna *et al.*, 1975). This posterior displacement is then spontaneously reduced as the neck is flexed (Marar, 1974).

There remain cases such as that reported by Scott where the lesion must be vascular, where infarction of the cord can occur without physical compromise of the capacity of the canal. Some of these patients die soon after injury from intracerebral bleeding or infarction and the state of the cervical cord is not adequately examined at post mortem. This central cervical lesion is perhaps more common than is

realized (Torg *et al.*, 1986). The damage may be sufficiently extensive to involve the brainstem and cranial nuclei (Hildingson *et al.*, 1989; Tamura, 1989).

Extension injuries of the neck in ankylosing spondylitis are even more dangerous. They are discussed in Chapter 8.

Acceleration flexion injuries

Acceleration/flexion will rotate the head and neck forwards until the chin strikes the chest. This range of movement is within normal limits and provided there is not already restricted movement due to degenerative change, no great damage will ensue.

Continuing forced flexion of the neck by the application of force to the vertex of the skull is of course the mechanism of injury in fracture dislocation, and is discussed in Chapter 4; but disruption of the posterior complex to a degree less extensive than that causing the 'hidden flexion' injury can occur. It is perhaps artificial to describe different degrees of severity of injury produced by the same mechanism as separate entities; but this group has sufficiently characteristic signs to merit discussion. These signs are:

1 Symptoms and signs of severe soft tissue sprain
2 No radiological evidence of bony damage
3 No radiological evidence of degenerative disease
4 Persistent alteration in the alignment of the flexed spine, but no isolated separation of spinous processes
5 Demonstrable evidence of multiple segment posterior soft tissue injury at operation.

The mechanism of such injury has been discussed, and it has been demonstrated experimentally that forward dislocation is the result of sagittal hyperflexion with added vertical load (Bauze and Ardran, 1978). Earlier experiments suggested that rotation was a necessary component in the production of dislocation, and that hyperflexion alone could not produce pure dislocation (Roaf, 1960).

The posterior soft tissue complex of the cervical spine is a poor relative of its lumbar counterpart. The ligamentum nuchae is strung between the vertebra prominens and the occiput without specific attachment to the individual spinous processes in between. The interspinous ligament hangs from it and the whole serves only as a septum providing origin for the trapezius and splenius muscles. The ligamentum flavum is the only strong and elastic structure behind the apophyseal joints. The capsules of these joints are richly innervated with proprioceptive and nociceptive receptors so that muscular control of neck stability is sensitive (Rissanen, 1960; Wyke, 1978).

The interpretation of flexion injuries in children is difficult as pseudo-subluxation is a normal radiological finding in a high proportion of children.

Lateral flexion acceleration injuries

Lateral flexion of the neck normally allows the ear to touch the shoulder. The movement is inevitably accompanied by rotation. The cord and nerve roots adapt to spinal canal movement by elastic deformation, while the dura concertinas on the concave side of movement. The locking mechanism of the apophyseal-transverse angle blocks lateral movement of the column before the nerve root sleeves and the vertebral artery are compromised. An unsustained lateral acceleration force is therefore expended within normal anatomical limits (Breig, 1960; McNab, 1964; Veleanu, 1975).

There are instances where lateral flexion is accompanied by forward flexion, so that the rotated head and neck are forced down in front of the shoulder. The shoulder away from the side of flexion may be forced down, as when a motor cyclist sustained a traction injury of the brachial plexus. Roaf (1963) described a series of cases in whom cervical injuries were associated with brachial plexus lesions (Roaf, 1963). The soft tissue lesion may be both posterior and lateral in such patients. The nerve root lesion may be central, as Sunderland (1974) has shown, when the force of injury is a combination of forward and lateral flexion. The dura in these circumstances remains intact. A lateral force alone is more likely to tear the dura before the nerve root is avulsed from the cord. The development of traumatic meningoceles following such injury may result in late onset signs of cord pressure appearing in patients with brachial plexus injuries. Three cases have been reported, and in two of them the presence of a soft tissue neck injury in addition to the brachial plexus lesion had been recognized from the onset (Pye and Hickey, 1975).

References

Babcock, J.L. (1976) Cervical spine injuries. *Archives of Surgery*, **111**, 646.

Bauze, R.J. and Ardran, G.M. (1978) Experimental production of forward dislocation in the human cervical spine. *Journal of Bone and Joint Surgery*, **60B**, 239.

Brain, Lord and Wilkinson, M. (1967) *Cervical Spondylosis and Other Disorders of the Spine.* London, Heinemann.

Breck, L.W. and Van Norman, R.W. (1971) Medicolegal aspects of cervical sprains. *Clinical Orthopaedics*, **74**, 124–128.

Breig, A. (1960) *Biomechanics of the Nervous System.* Stockholm. Almquist and Wiksell. p. 31.

Burke, D.C. (1971) Hyperextension injuries of the spine. *Journal of Bone and Joint Surgery*, **53B**, 3.

Burrows, E.H. (1963) Sagittal diameters of the spinal cord in cervical spondylosis. *Clinical Radiology*, **14**, 77.

Crowe, H.E. (1928) Injuries to the cervical spine. Presented to *Annual Meeting of Western Orthopaedic Association.* San Francisco.

Deans, G.T., Magalliard, J.N., Kerr, M. and Rutherford, W.H. (1987) Neck sprain. *Injury*, **18**, 10.

Edwards, W.C. and La Rocca, H. (1983) Developmental sagittal diameter of cervical canal. *Spine*, **8**, 20.

Ehni, G. (1984) Biomechanics of the cervical spine. In *Cervical Arthroses.* Chicago, Year Book Med. Publ. Inc. p. 78.

Friedenberg, Z.B. and Miller, W.I. (1963) Degenerative disc disease of the cervical spine. *Journal of Bone and Joint Surgery*, **45A**, 1171.

Gotten, N. (1956) Surgery of one hundred cases of whiplash injury after settlement of injury. *Journal of the American Medical Association*, **162**, 865.

Greenfield, J. and Illfield, F.W. (1977) Acute cervical strain. *Clinical Orthopaedics*, **122**, 196.

Gupta, A. (1987) Anterior fusion for cervical disc disease. *M. Ch. Orth. Thesis*, University of Liverpool.

Hildingson, C., Wenngren, B.I., Bring, G. and Toolanan, G. (1989) Oculomotor problems after acute cervical spine injury. *Acta Orthopaedica Scandinavica*, **60**, 513.

Hodge, J.R. (1971) The whiplash neurosis. *Psychosomatics*, **12**, 245.

Hodgson, S.P. and Grundy, M. (1989) Whiplash injuries: their long term prognosis and its relationship to compensation. *Neuro-orthopaedics*, **7**, 88–89.

Hohl, M. (1974) Soft tissue injuries of the neck in automobile accidents. *Journal of Bone and Joint Surgery*, **56A**, 1675.

Hohl, M. (1975) Soft tissue injuries of the neck. *Clinical Orthopaedics and Related Research*, **109**, 42–49.

Howcroft, A.J. and Jenkins, D.H.R. (1977) Potentially fatal asphyxia following minor injury of cervical spine. *Journal of Bone and Joint Surgery*, **59B**, 93.

Jeffreys, T.E. (1991) *Prognosis in Musculo-Skeletal Injury*. Oxford, Butterworth Heinemann. p. 24.

Johnson, R.M., Hart, D.L., Simmons, E.F., Ramsby, G.R. and Southwick, J.O. (1977) Cervical orthoses, a comparative study. *Journal of Bone and Joint Surgery*, **59A**, 332–339.

Knapper, W.A. (1964) Whiplash injury–not a diagnosis. *The Defence Research Institute.* Milwaukee.

McNab, I. (1964) Acceleration injuries of the cervical spine. *Journal of Bone and Joint Surgery*, **46A**, 1797.

McNab, I. (1971) The whiplash syndrome. *Orthopedic Clinics of North America*, **2**, 389.

McNab, I. (1973) The whiplash syndrome. *Clinical Neurosurgery*, **20**, 232.

Marar, B.C. (1974) Hyperextension injuries of cervical spine. *Journal of Bone and Joint Surgery*, **56A**, 1655.

Norris, S.H. and Watt, I. (1983) The prognosis of neck injuries resulting from rearend vehicle collisions. *Journal of Bone and Joint Surgery*, **65B**, 608.

Pallis, C., Jones, A.M. and Spillane, A.D. (1954) Cervical spondylosis, incidence and implications. *Brain*, **77**, 274.

Perna, E., Petrone, G. and Liguori, R. (1975) Tetraplegia from trauma in absence of fractures and luxations. *Journal of Neurological Sciences*, **19**, 171.

Pye, I.F. and Hickey, M.C. (1975) Traumatic arachnoid diverticula causing cord compression. *British Journal of Radiology*, **48**, 889.

Rissanen, P.M. (1960) Anatomy of supraspinatus ligaments. *Acta Orthopaedica Scandinavica*, Suppl. 46.

Roaf, R. (1960) A study of the mechanics of spinal injuries. *Journal of Bone and Joint Surgery*, **42B**, 810–823.

Roaf, R. (1963) Lateral flexion injury of the cervical spine. *Journal of Bone and Joint Surgery*, **45B**, 36.

Scott, P.J. (1963) Delayed traumatic paraplegia. *Journal of Bone and Joint Surgery*, **45B**, 719.

Sunderland, S. (1974) Mechanism of cervical nerve root evulsion in injuries of neck and shoulder. *Journal of Neurosurgery*, **41**, 705.

Tamura, T. (1989) Cranial symptoms after cervical injury. *Journal of Bone and Joint Surgery*, **71B**, 283.

Taylor, A.R. (1951) The mechanism of injury to the spinal cord in the neck. *Journal of Bone and Joint Surgery*, **33B**, 543.

Taylor, A.R. and Blackwood, W. (1948) Paraplegia in hyperextension. *Journal of Bone and Joint Surgery*, **30B**, 245.

Tokarz, F. and Stachowski, B. (1974) Trauma of cervical vertebral column complicated by vertebral artery insufficiency. *Patologia Polska*, **25**, 445.

Torg, J.S., Pavlov, H., Gennaro, S. *et al.* (1986) Neuropraxia of the cervical spinal cord. *Journal of Bone and Joint Surgery*, **68A**, 1355.

Veleanu, C. (1975) The cervical locking mechanism. *Morphology and Embryology*, **21**, 3–7.

Watson-Jones, R. (1940) *Fractures and Joint Injuries*. Edinburgh, Livingstone.

Weir, D.C. (1975) Roentgenographic signs of cervical injury. *Clinical Orthopaedics*, **109**, 9–17.

Wickstrom, J. and La Rocca, H. (1974) Management of cervical spine injuries from acceleration forces. *Current Practice in Orthopaedic Surgery*, 83–98.

Wickstrom, J., Rodriguez, R. and Martinez, J. (1968) Experimental production of acceleration injuries of head and neck. *Accident Pathology*, Washington, DC: US Printing Office.

Wyke, B. (1978) Clinical significance of articular receptor systems. *Annals of the Royal College of Surgeons of England*, **60**, 137.

Zatskin, H.R. and Kreton, F. (1961) Evaluation of the cervical spine in whiplash injuries. *Radiology*, **75**, 577.

7 Cervical spondylosis

Time's on the wing
Life never knows the return of Spring.

John Gay (1782)
The Beggars Opera.

Introduction

The radiographic changes of cervical spondylosis are present in more than 80 per cent of people over the age of 55 years (Brain, 1962). These changes, once present, do not necessarily progress (Pallis, Jones and Spillane, 1954). If unselected patients over the age of 50, admitted to hospital with symptoms unrelated to the central nervous system are examined, signs of cervical cord or cervical root lesions will be found in many. There is an association between the signs thus found, and the radiographic appearances of the cervical spine (Pallis, Jones and Spillane, 1954). The structural changes seen on radiographs, can exist without producing any symptoms or signs. Although the radiographic appearances are universal in the aged, the incidence of serious complaints due to cervical spondylosis is low. But episodic neck pain is probably as universal as the radiographic change. The clinical syndromes of cervical spondylosis cannot be explained only in terms of structural degeneration. Other factors in the aetiology of the clinical picture include trauma, ischaemia and congenital narrowing of the spinal canal.

The structural changes associated with ageing

The radiographic changes of cervical spondylosis are those of the bony skeleton. They are:

1 Narrowing of the intervertebral disc space.
2 Osteophyte formation at the margins of the vertebral bodies.
3 Sclerosis beneath the vertebral end plate.
4 Osteophyte formation adjacent to the neurocentral lip.
5 Narrowing of the apophyseal joint spaces with osteophyte formation at the margins of the facets (Figures 7.1, 7.2, 7.3).

These bony changes follow desiccation of the intervertebral disc and osteoarthrosis of the posterior joints. Ageing also affects the supporting soft tissue structures of the spine.

The intervertebral discs of the cervical spine are limited laterally by the neurocentral lips of the vertebral bodies. In the adult spine clefts are apparent in the lateral margins of the disc between the neurocentral lip and the adjacent groove of the vertebra above. These develop in the normal disc in the second decade of life. They are fissures in the annulus of the disc, formed by loosening of the more peripheral lamellae and lateral bulging of the inner lamellae. The fissures remain closed laterally and extend medially into the nucleus of the disc. The peripheral layers undergo metaplasia to simulate capsular connective tissue. The outer layer may erode and the nucleus communicate with the intervertebral foramen. Desiccation of the disc leads to fibrosis and the bulging annulus now forms the outer 'capsule' of the neurocentral 'joint'. In the lower cervical vertebrae these 'joints' assume the load carrying functions of the disc itself. These segments,

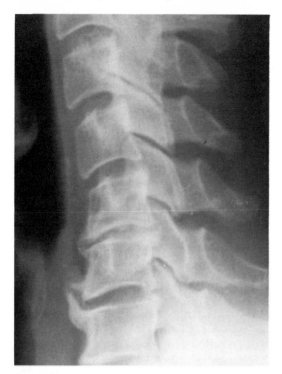

Figure 7.1. Cervical spondylosis, lateral view.

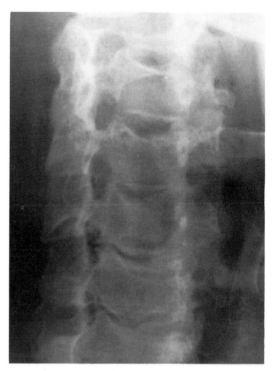

Figure 7.3. Cervical spondylosis, oblique view, showing encroachment on intervertebral foramina.

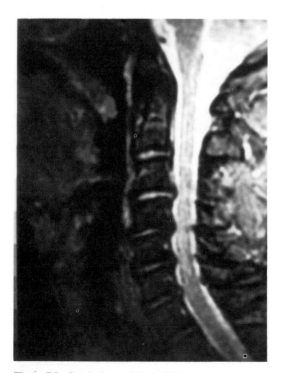

Figure 7.2. Cervical spondylosis. MRI.

C5/6 and C6/7, are also those where most movement occurs. The three prerequisites of osteoarthrosis – age, weight-bearing and movement – now exist, and the neurocentral 'joint' responds accordingly with osteophytic lipping and subchondral sclerosis. As the degenerating disc loses height, the proliferative swelling of the neurocentral lip protrudes into the intervertebral foramen.

The nucleus of the disc in youth has the capacity to retain and discharge water diurnally, a phenomenon it shares with all connective tissue. There is a close correlation between water content and elasticity of the disc. The ratio of the water content of the nucleus to that of the annulus remains approximately equal until the fifth decade when rapid desiccation occurs in the nucleus (Saunders and Inman, 1939; Wilkinson, 1960; Freidenberg and Miller, 1963; Boden *et al.*, 1990).

Similar bulging of the disc, accompanied by spondylotic lipping, occurs anteriorly. The anterior longitudinal ligament, weakly attached already to the annulus, becomes stretched and vulnerable to minor injury.

Posterior bulging of the annulus and the osteophytes that follow form the familiar spondylotic ridges that encroach on the spinal canal.

The changes in the disc are the primary lesion in cervical spondylosis. The structural changes in bone and in associated structures are the precipitating lesions of the clinical syndromes which result (Boni and Denaro, 1987).

The apophyseal joints of the lower cervical spine are less often affected by osteoarthrosis than those of the upper segments. The disc changes are more pronounced in the lower cervical segments, and apophyseal movements at these levels are correspondingly reduced. Yet the loss of disc height must lead to a degree of apophyseal subluxation. The discrepancy in distribution of posterior osteoarthrosis between upper and lower cervical segments has not been adequately explained (Bowden, 1966; Holt and Yates, 1966; Hirsch, Schajowitz and Galante, 1967; Sager, 1972; Tondbury, 1972).

There is no disc between atlas and axis but the synovial joints between the two vertebrae are commonly affected by osteoarthrosis (Benner and Ehni, 1983).

The ligamentum flavum buckles and becomes hypertrophied as the laminae overlap with loss of disc height. This further diminishes the capacity of the spinal canal.

The dura corrugates and unfolds during flexion and extension of the spine. If spondylotic ridges press on it, it tends to remain corrugated. Thickening of the dentate ligaments further tethers the dura. This thickening is not uniform and lesions in the spinal cord appear to be related to areas of dentate ligament thickening (Bedford, Bosanquet and Russell, 1952; Brain and Wilkinson, 1967). The anchoring effect of the dentate ligaments is also said to be one of the reasons why the spinal cord is more vulnerable to sagittal rather than coronal squeeze (Kahn, 1947; Rogers, 1961). The dura blends with the nerve roots in the intervertebral foramina, and if it is corrugated the nerve roots are anchored during extension of the spine. The spondylotic projections of the neurocentral lip compromise the capacity of the intervertebral funnel and provoke an inflammatory response in the connective tissue surrounding the root sleeves. The consequent fibrosis will further tether the dura, and the nerve roots and radicular vessels will be stretched during neck movement. The posterior root ganglion lies above the anterior root in the funnel and is more often affected by encroachment of the neurocentral and apophyseal osteophytes. The anterior root tucks itself out of harms way underneath the overhang (Abdullah, 1958).

The histological changes in *the nerve roots* are fibrosis of nerve sheaths with patchy axonal and myelin degeneration. These changes are thought to be secondary to the root sleeve fibrosis described above and are probably caused by radicular arterial ischaemia (Holt and Yates, 1966; Brain and Wilkinson, 1967; Olssen, Sourander and Kristensen, 1972).

The sagittal diameter of the spinal canal

There is a relationship between the sagittal diameter of the spinal canal and cervical myelopathy. Sagittal compression is more likely to damage the cord than coronal compression (Doppman, 1975; Gooding, Wilson and Hoff, 1975). Soft tissue structures such as disc protrusions and corrugations of the dura and ligamentum flavum, can increase compression (Wilkinson, 1960). Malformation of the cord corresponds with spondylotic ridges (Hughes, 1978). Compression can occur in Paget's disease (Curran, 1975) and in ossification of the posterior longitudinal ligament (Nagashima, 1972; Nakanishi *et al.*, 1974).

The mechanism of cord damage is a mixture of direct neural compression and arterial ischaemia from stretching of laterally transverse arteries in the central grey matter. The sagittal diameter of the canal at the level of C3 varies between 15 and 20 mm. It then remains constant to C7 (Burrows, 1963). It can be measured on standard lateral radiographs between the posterior margin of the vertebral body and the spinolaminar line (Tchang, 1974) (Figure 7.4). These measurements however apply only to the bony skeleton and calcified tissues such as spondylotic disc protrusions. The enhanced imaging of CT and MRI also shows soft tissue changes.

Blood supply

Atherosclerosis of the vertebral arteries is a common finding in old age (Hutchinson and

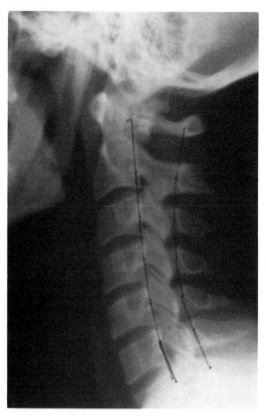

Figure 7.4. Sagittal diameters in the cervical spine.

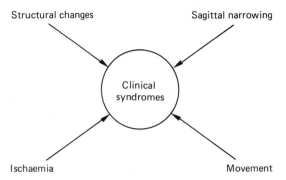

Figure 7.5. Factors involved in producing a clinical syndrome.

Yates, 1956). It may contribute to the ischaemia of nerve roots and cord already produced by the fibrotic constriction of the radicular and medullary feeder branches in the intervertebral foramen. Even in the absence of atherosclerosis, but more so if it is present, the second part of the artery is vulnerable as it passes immediately lateral to the neurocentral lip (Hardin, 1963; Nagashima, 1970; Smith, Vanderark and Kempe, 1971). The trauma of acceleration extension injury, or the repeated trauma of occupation may compromise the artery in the spondylotic neck (Tokay and Stachowski, 1974). The effects of disturbing the vertebrobasilar circulation can vary from transient dizziness to infarction of the medulla and cerebellum.

Trauma

A single episode of injury can be responsible for an acute cervical disc prolapse in a previously healthy cervical spine. This is uncommon. More commonly a neck injury in someone who already has cervical spondylosis can trigger a cervical disc syndrome, radiculopathy, myelopathy or vertebrobasilar syndrome. This neck injury can be isolated or the repetitive injury of chronic occupational trauma. Occupational injury was recognized as associated with disc disease during the last century (Lane, 1886). The mechanism by which trauma can trigger a clinical syndrome is conjectural in most cases; but stretching of ligaments and fibrotic nerve roots, bulging inwards of ligamentum flavum, microfractures, extra-dural haemorrhages, infarction of nerve roots or cord, are all possible.

These factors, and their part in producing a clinical picture can be represented diagramatically as shown in Figure 7.5. They all stem from degeneration of the intervertebral disc.

The clinical syndromes associated with cervical spondylosis

Brain and Wilkinson (1967) grouped their patients according to their symptoms:

1 Acute radiculopathy–first onset acute and acute on chronic.
2 Chronic radiculopathy.
3 Cervical myelopathy.
4 Patients presenting with pain in the neck.
5 Patients presenting with headache.
6 Patients with symptoms of vertebrobasilar ischaemia.

A simpler classification is:

1 Acute cervical disc prolapse.
2 Chronic radiculopathy and the 'cervical disc syndrome'.
3 Cervical myelopathy.
4 Vertebrobasilar disease.

1 Acute prolapse of a cervical disc

These patients can present with no previous history of pain in the neck or arm, or the acute episode may occur against a chronic background. There may be a history of previous lumbar disc problems. There may or may not be a history of injury. The injury can occur weeks or months before the onset of acute symptoms.

The patient will present with pain in the neck, radiating into the dermatome supplied by the affected nerve root. Pain in the neck may be the more prominent feature, with paraesthesia or numbness in the relevant dermatome. There may be appropriate reflex loss or motor weakness. Over 80 per cent of acute prolapses involve the sixth or seventh cervical roots. The sensory symptoms therefore will be felt in the thumb, index and middle fingers. The pain will be aggravated by coughing. The biceps and supinator jerks may be lost. Motor weakness can affect elbow flexion, forearm rotation and wrist flexion and extension. Neck movements will be restricted and painful and the head and neck may be held tilted towards the side of the lesion.

The pain felt in the arm must be differentiated from the pain of nerve root and peripheral nerve compression from other causes. Destructive lesions of the neck such as tumour must be excluded as must compressive neuropathies of peripheral nerves. The common carpal tunnel syndrome is to be considered in the differential diagnosis of a chronic disc lesion but can hardly be confused with the acute picture of an acutely prolapsed cervical disc.

Standard radiographs will serve to exclude destructive lesions. They may or may not show spondylosis. Whether they do or not depends on the age of the patient. An epidemiological study has shown the male to female ratio as being 1.4 to 1.0, and maximal frequency in the fourth and fifth decades (Kelsey, Gittens and Walter, 1984).

The initial management of acute prolapse is conservative and there is no need at this stage to investigate further unless sophisticated imaging facilities are immediately available. Thorough clinical examination and standard radiography should establish a firm diagnosis of disc prolapse. Clinical examination has a high ability to predict the correct level, as a review of studies, carried out before modern methods of imaging existed, demonstrated (Yoss *et al.*, 1957).

The principles of treatment at this stage are rest and analgesia. A well-fitting collar relieves neck pain even if it is not mechanically efficient (see Chapter 5). Strong analgesia may be necessary.

Failure to relieve pain, and a persisting or progressing neurological defect are indications for operation. The neck should not be manipulated. At this stage precise localization of the prolapse is required and cervical radiculography, CT scanning or MRI will provide this (Figure 7.6).

Cervical disc prolapse can be approached via the posterior approach (foraminotomy) or anteriorly. The use of the microscope is an advantage in both procedures. Microsurgical foraminotomy aims to decompress the nerve root by excising the posterior and inferior walls of the intervertebral foramen without disturbing the disc prolapse (Williams, 1983).

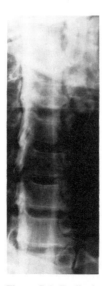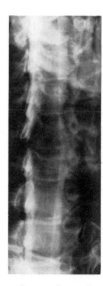

Figure 7.6. Radiculogram of acute disc prolapse at C6/7.

Good results are claimed but extruded disc fragments are left in place.

Microsurgical anterior discectomy allows thorough clearance of the disc space and removal of extruded disc fragments within the canal and foramen. Fusion is said not to be necessary after this procedure (Martins, 1976).

The acute stiff neck is a condition more familiar to family doctors and osteopaths than orthopaedic surgeons or neurosurgeons – unless they have suffered from it themselves. The patient is usually a young adult in good health. There is no history of injury. There is no history of previous neck or arm pain. There is sudden onset of severe neck pain, perhaps when waking. The head is held in a fixed position, usually tilted. Movement is absent in one direction, restricted in others. There is no radiation of pain. There is no giddiness. There are no abnormal neurological signs in the arms or the legs. Radiographs of the neck are uninformative.

If the patient is seen quickly, strong manual traction will abolish the pain. There are certain absolute contraindications to this manoeuvre. It must never be used in a child. Acute torticollie in a child may be due to atlanto-axial subluxation (Watson-Jones, 1932; Dewar *et al.*, 1964). It must not be used after injury or when there are any abnormal neurological signs.

2 Chronic radiculopathy and the cervical disc syndrome

Pain in the neck, with or without radiation of the pain into the shoulders and arms or up into the back of the head is as common a presenting symptom in orthopaedic clinics as is low back pain. When the pain is due to the compression of a nerve root in the intervertebral foramen by the structural changes of cervical spondylosis, it will be felt in the relevant dermatomes of the compressed roots. Pain in the neck itself, or in the back of the head, will arise from osteoarthritic apophyseal joints, more so in the upper cervical spine, and from radiation into the dermatomes of the upper cervical nerves. Pain can also arise from the annulus of the disc and the supporting ligaments of the affected segments. This pain is mediated by the sinuvertebral nerve. It will be experienced in the sclerotome of the affected segment (Kellgren, 1939). This pain differs from radicular pain in that it is deeper, poorly localized and more diffuse. It is described as being dull and burning – very different from the sharp pain and tingling of radiculopathy. It will be felt in areas that have no neurological relation with the affected segment – for example, it can be felt between the shoulder blades in lower cervical lesions, or affect areas of the upper limb not innervated by any specific nerve root.

More than one cervical segment may be a source of pain. The radicular and discogenic elements may contribute disproportionately at different levels. One element may predominate. The symptoms may vary in type, distribution and intensity.

The natural history of chronic cervical disc disease is, on the whole, benign. Symptoms persist intermittently for years with periods of remission and relapse occurring either with or without the precipitation of injury. The radiographic appearances slowly deteriorate, but there is no correlation between clinical and radiographic progress.

Differential diagnosis is not difficult in the majority. A complete neurological examination is essential when each patient is first seen. If long tract signs are found in the lower limbs, the symptoms and signs in the upper limbs are likely to be also due to lesions in the cord itself (Phillips, 1975).

Problems can arise when the presenting symptom is of pain and paraesthesia in the arm only. The classical carpal tunnel syndrome is easy enough to recognize, as is classical ulnar neuritis at the elbow, but proximal spread of pain in these syndromes does occur. Barton (1987) states that pain felt in the back of the hand is more likely to be of cervical origin. That is not my experience. Cervical disc lesions and carpal tunnel syndromes may coexist (Murray-Leslie and Wright, 1976). Conduction studies may help to establish the clinically dominant lesion.

Compression syndromes at the thoracic outlet should not cause undue difficulty in diagnosis. They are rare. The radiographic finding of a cervical rib is irrelevant, but there may be a fibrous band extending down to the first rib. If this does cause symptoms the lowest cervical roots will be involved and the small muscles of the hand will be affected first (Gilliatt, 1979; King and Bonney, 1983).

Dysphagia can be caused by prominent anterior osteophytes at the C5/6 and C6/7 levels. The symptom may be sufficiently troublesome to justify operative excision. The operation must include excision of the disc and fusion of the segment, otherwise the osteophytes will recur (Stuart, 1975, 1989).

Management of the chronic cervical disc syndrome must be based on the understanding that it is a chronic, painful but benign condition which pursues a course of remission and relapse. In many patients the symptoms are aggravated by anxiety. Frank discussion of the natural history once the diagnosis has been established will not only alleviate fears but prevent disappointment if relapse occurs after apparently successful treatment. If the neck has been injured at work or in a road accident, the prognosis can be influenced adversely (see Chapter 6).

Treatment, then, is directed towards the relief of pain, while awaiting natural remission. The chances of resolution are high so every type of treatment from acupuncture to Zen meditation will have a high rate of success. Commonsense dictates that treatment must not be harmful. Muscle spasm responds to rest. A programme of splintage with a collar, analgesics and a course of exercises once the pain has settled is effective and simple.

The pain may be so severe in some patients that bed rest and heavy analgesia are required. Such patients must be carefully observed as they may have developed an acute disc prolapse.

A minority of patients remain with intractable pain or with recurrences so frequent and severe as to interfere with their everyday life. They must be considered for treatment by operation.

The indication for operation is pain. The pain may be radicular in origin, discogenic, or both. Rarely does a progressive lower motor neurone lesion make operation imperative. Pain is a complex experience; it has an affective component and is difficult to assess objectively. It is influenced by personality, by environment, by emotion. Attempts have been made to measure it by mapping areas of decreased electrical resistance in affected areas, but the results were inconclusive (Riley and Richter, 1975). The decision to operate must be a joint decision between surgeon and patient. The surgeon is entitled to advise the

advantages of an operation against a possible prolonged natural history (Green, 1977). He owes it to himself as well as to his patient, if he feels that operation is not indicated for reasons other than physical, to refuse to operate.

The objective of the operation is to remove the source of the pain. This source must be identified before any operation is planned or advised.

The source of pain may be a compressed nerve root or it may be a degenerate disc alone. There may be more than one source of pain, at more than one level. There is no correlation between plain radiographs and the clinical picture, and other investigations are necessary.

The dimensions of the canal and the intervertebral foramina can be shown by radiculography. The definition with water soluble contrast media is excellent and the investigation is safe. Computed tomography, with or without contrast, will show transverse axial dimensions and reconstruction will demonstrate abnormalities in the sagittal plane. Magnetic resonance imaging demonstrates abnormalities of the disc and cord but does not clearly define root problems.

A disc may be identified as a source of pain by provocative discography. The disc is injected with a fluid – using a contrast medium confirms the level and shows the morphology of the disc. This injection is painful. If the pain is similar to the pain usually felt by the patient, and if it is immediately abolished by the injection of a local anaesthetic, it can be inferred that that disc is a source of pain. Any morphological abnormalities, such as leakage of the medium through the neurocentral lips can be ignored as being as irrelevant as the degenerative changes seen on the standard films (Figure 7.7) (Holt, 1964; Kikuchi, McNab and Moreau, 1981; Whitecloud and Seago, 1987).

We have reviewed my patients investigated by discography and subsequently treated by anterior interbody fusion. Two hundred and thirty-four discs were injected in 90 patients. Of these discs 130 were subsequently excised and the segments fused. Where discography identified a pain source, immediate pain relief was experienced in 89.9 per cent of cases. In these same patients excellent and good results at one year persisted in 77.7 per cent. Poor results were found when more discs than pain

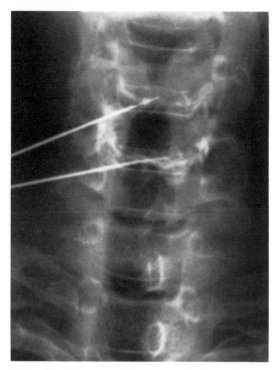

Figure 7.7. Discogram of degenerate disc showing leakage of contrast medium.

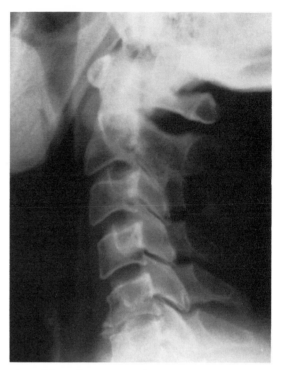

Figure 7.9. Collapse of graft (and recurrence of symptoms) 7 weeks after operation.

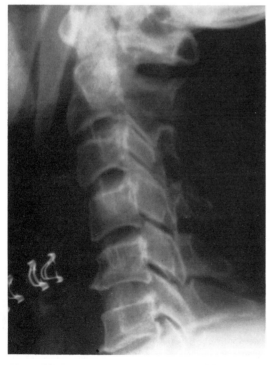

Figure 7.8. Interbody autogenous grafts at C5/6 and C6/7.

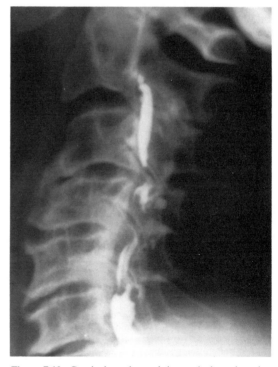

Figure 7.10. Cervical myelograph in cervical myelopathy.

sources were excised, and when fusion did not occur (Gupta, 1987).

The grafts used in these patients were autogenous, obtained from the crest of the ilium (Figure 7.8). This donor site can be a postoperative nuisance (Summers and Eisenstein, 1989). Allografts avoid this complication, but they do not resist compression as well as autografts (Figure 7.9). Bone substitutes are now available commercially.

3 Cervical myelopathy

The clinical picture of cervical myelopathy can be explained on the anatomical distribution of the lesions within the spinal cord. There is demyelination of the lateral column at the level of the lesion which usually corresponds to the level of the spondylotic ridge indenting the cord (and may therefore be multisegmental), with degeneration of the anterior parts of the posterior column and destruction of the central grey matter. The degeneration of the posterior (afferent) columns will extend upwards, that of the descending lateral columns downwards. The grey matter necrosis may extend upwards for a short distance (Wilkinson, 1960; Hughes, 1978). Accurate clinical localization of the level of involvement is therefore difficult. The initial presentation may be of a lower lesion (Mair and Duckman, 1953; Taylor and Byrnes, 1974).

Examination of elderly people without neurological symptoms will often disclose signs of long tract involvement and it is possible that many cases never present clinically (Pallis, Jones and Spillane, 1954). The typical clinical picture is that of a man (more often than a woman) aged over 50, who has spent his working life in hard manual labour, complaining of the gradual onset of weakness in his legs. He very often gives a history of injury following which his symptoms began (Gupta, 1987). He will often complain of pain and stiffness in his neck, perhaps radiating into his shoulders and arms with tingling in his fingers. Pain in the legs is not a common presenting symptom.

Examination at this time may or may not demonstrate limited neck movement (Clarke and Robinson, 1956). Examination of the legs will show spasticity, brisk reflexes, clonus and perhaps extensor plantar responses. Standard radiographs of the neck will always reveal narrowing of the disc spaces and osteophyte formation, at one or more levels, the C5/6 level being the most commonly and most severely involved (Figure 7.10). At the level of these spondylotic ridges the sagittal diameter of the canal is reduced. Measurement of the depth from the middle of the vertebral body may well show that the canal is developmentally shallow. Attempts have been made to give numerical values to these measurements but this is an academic exercise. Those interested will find details in several papers (Payne and Spillane, 1957; Burrows, 1963; Edwards and La Rocca, 1983; Torg *et al.*, 1986; Matsuma *et al.*, 1989).

The natural history is unpredictable except that progress will be slow. The usual pattern is one of episodic attacks each leaving a slowly increasing residual defect. There is never complete remission of signs. A minority, about one fifth, continue to deteriorate steadily until spastic paraplegia or even tetraplegia develops. A small minority retain, without further loss, the neurological defect found on first examination.

The presence of 'cervical root' symptoms and signs in the arms can be confusing. The question arises whether there are two distinct compressive lesions, one in the foramen and one in the canal or whether the whole picture is myelopathic. Consensus favours the latter (Phillips, 1975; Gregorius, Estrin and Crandall, 1976). Some other symptoms can also confuse. The radiation of pain into the head, dysphagia, vertigo and ataxia may be due to associated vertebrobasilar ischaemia or they can be due to involvement of the relevant spinal tracts. 'Drop' attacks are usually due to cerebral ischaemia but have been reported as having been caused by cervical disc prolapse (Maurice-Williams, 1974). Coccydynia has been blamed on cervical myelopathy (Kobayashi, 1974). 'Searching movements', or pseudo-athetosis, due to posterior column loss, are described (Bickerstaff, 1978, personal communication). Impotence is a common symptom (Schneider, 1974). Bladder sphincter dysfunction is present in many patients but is not necessarily a sign of severe myelopathy as bladder neck obstruction from prostatism is common in elderly men. The non-specific Lhermitte phenomenon when movements of the head and neck produce electric shock like feelings spreading throughout the body signifies a severe myelopathy and a poor prognosis (Gregorius, Estrin and Crandall, 1976; Gupta, 1987).

The differential diagnosis includes other compressive lesions of the cervical canal, such as congenital malformations and tumours (Taylor and Byrnes, 1974), and multiple sclerosis. This affects younger patients, tends to be more abrupt in onset and can remit completely. In cervical myelopathy complete remission never occurs.

The management of cervical myelopathy is expectant. Symptoms are eased by the provision of a collar. If neurological deterioration continues, consideration must be given to operative intervention. If operation is considered it should be done before significant disability has occurred (Jeffreys, 1986).

Posterior operations were the first used. Laminectomy is carried out from one level above and one level below the involved segments. In practice, this means decompression from C3 to C7. Laminectomy is still used with good effect in selected cases, particularly when the sagittal squeeze is produced by thickening of the ligamentum flavum (Jeffreys, 1979).

Anterior decompression is used, with or without fusion. An argument in favour of fusion is that if subsequent laminectomy should prove necessary, the spine will not become unstable (Uttley and Monro, 1989).

4 Vertebrobasilar disease

In 1897 Wallenberg described two cases of unilateral infarction of the lateral aspect of the medulla and the inferior aspect of the cerebellum (Figure 7.11). Both cases were caused by occlusion of the posterior inferior cerebellar artery. It has since been recognized that disease of the vertebral arteries is more often responsible for the syndrome (Wallenberg, 1897; Quast and Liebegott, 1975). Most cases occur on the left side. This may be due to the left vertebral artery being the larger or even the only vessel. For an unknown reason, vertebral artery thrombosis in women taking the contraceptive pill is more common on the right side (Ask-Upmark and Bickerstaff, 1976).

Vertebral artery ischaemia is the main cause of Wallenberg or lateral medullary syndrome. The second part of the vertebral artery is vulnerable to distortion by osteophytes in cervical spondylosis (Hutchinson and Yates, 1956). The pathology is considered to be progressive stenosis of an already atherosclerotic vessel from thrombosis or occlusion from without, but embolism of the posterior cerebral artery has been described (McEwan, 1967; Sullivan *et al.*, 1975). A case has been reported in a child (Klein, Snyder and Schwartz, 1976). The third part of the vertebral artery follows a tortuous line from the axis to its entrance into the extradural space.

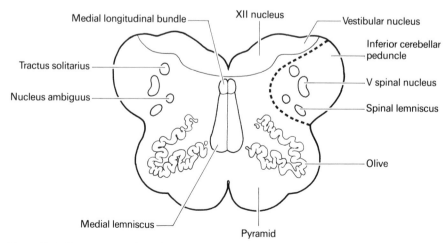

Figure 7.11. Transverse section of medulla. The dotted line encloses the area infarcted by occlusion of the posterior inferior cerebellar artery.

In rotation of the head and neck to one side the contralateral artery is stretched and the ipsilateral vessel compressed. Extension of the head can also interfere with flow. A case has been reported of lateral medullary syndrome in a man who spent two days painting his ceiling (Okawara and Nibbelink, 1974). Fortunately for posterity Michelangelo and Maulperstch painted their respective ceilings lying flat on their backs. The vertebral artery may be damaged during manipulation of the neck (Davidson, Welford and Dixon, 1975). Vertebral angiography may dislodge atheromatous plaques and thrombi (Brown, 1976).

Vertebral artery disease can be responsible for a wide range of clinical conditions ranging from transient attacks of vertigo, associated with head and neck movement, to the fully developed lateral medullary syndrome (Brain, 1962). The syndrome consists of most or all of the following features:

1 Vertigo and vomiting, often of acute onset.
2 Incoordination and ataxia on the side of the lesion.
3 Dysthesia, often described as a feeling of hot water running down the face, in the trigeminal area of the Vth nerve.
4 Dysphagia and palatal weakness on the affected side (damage to nerves IX and X in the nucleus ambiguus).
5 Altered pain and temperature appreciation on the opposite side of the body.
6 Horner's syndrome on the affected side.

Vertebrobasilar disease may coexist with cervical myelopathy which will confuse the neurological picture.

Management of the condition is expectant. Simple splintage of the neck may relieve symptoms of mild disease. Anticoagulation may be necessary. The artery is usually involved at several levels and there is associated generalized atherosclerosis. Direct surgical attack is unrewarding unless the lesion is limited to one or two segments. Decompression operations have been described (Hardin, 1963; Verbiest, 1968).

Operations on the cervical spine are dangerous. The incidence of complications is low in skilled hands; but they can be catastrophic. Neurological defects, even tetraplegia, cerebrovascular catastrophes and death have all been reported (Gregory, 1964; Flynn, 1982).

The indications must be clear and the surgical competence high before any of these procedures are attempted.

References

Abdullah, S. (1958) M.Sc. Thesis, quoted by Bowden (1966).

Ask-Upmark, O. and Bickerstaff, E. (1976) Vertebral artery occlusion and oral contraceptives. *British Medical Journal*, **1**, 487.

Barton, N. (1987) Upper limb problems. In *Neuromuscular Problems in Orthopaedics*. (Galasko, C.S.B., ed.) Oxford, Blackwells. p. 218.

Bedford, P.D., Bosanquet, F.D. and Russell, W.R. (1952) The dentate ligaments in cervical spondylosis. *Lancet*, **ii**, 55.

Benner, B.G. and Ehni, G.E. (1983) *Orthopaedic Transactions*, **7**, 121–124.

Boden, S.D., McCowin, P.R., Davis, D.O., Thomas, S.D., Mark, A.S. and Wiesel, S. (1990) Abnormal M.R. scans of cervical spine in asymptomatic subjects. *Journal of Bone and Joint Surgery*, **72A**, 1178.

Boni, M. and Denaro, V. (1987) Anatomo-clinical correlations in cervical spondylosis. *Cervical Spine*, **1**, 4.

Bowden, R.E.M. (1966) The applied anatomy of the cervical spine. *Proceedings of the Royal Society of Medicine*, **59**, 1142.

Brain, Lord (1962) Some unsolved problems in cervical spondylosis. *Gowers Memorial Lecture*. Royal College of Physicians, London.

Brain, Lord and Wilkinson, M. (1967) *Cervical Spondylosis*. London, Heinemann.

Brown, A.H. (1976) Medicolegal implications of angiography. *Radiologic Technology*, **47**, 252.

Burrows, E.H. (1963) Sagittal diameter of the spinal cord in cervical spondylosis. *Clinical Radiology*, **14**, 77.

Clarke, E. and Robinson, P.K. (1956) Cervical myelopathy: a complication of cervical spondylosis. *Brain*, **79**, 483.

Curran, J.E. (1975) Neurological sequelae of Paget's disease of vertebral column. *Australian Radiology*, **21**, 15.

Davidson, K.C., Welford, E.C. and Dixon, C.D. (1975) Traumatic vertebral artery pseudo-aneurysm after chiropractic manipulation. *Radiology*, **115**, 651.

Dewar, F.P., Duckworth, J.W., Wright, T.J. and Worsman, G. (1964) Subluxation of atlanto-axial joint in rotation. *Journal of Bone and Joint Surgery*, **46B**, 778.

Doppman, J.L. (1975) Ischaemia in antero-posterior compression of the cord. *Investigative Radiology*, **10**, 544.

Edwards, W.C. and La Rocca, H. (1983) Developmental sagittal diameter of cervical canal. *Spine*, **8**, 20.

Flynn, T.B. (1982) Neurologic complications of anterior cervical fusion. *Spine*, **7**, 536.

Freidenberg, Z.B. and Miller, W.T. (1963) Degenerative disc disease of the cervical spine. *Journal of Bone and Joint Surgery*, **45A**, 1171.

Gilliatt, R.W. (1979) The classical neurological syndrome

associated with a cervical rib and band. In *Pain in the Shoulder and Arm: an Integrated View*. (J.M. Greep, H.A.J. Lemmens, D.B. Roos and H.C. Urschel, eds.) The Hague, Martinus Nijhoff.

Gooding, M.R., Wilson, C.B. and Hoff, J.T. (1975) Experimental cervical myelopathy. *Surgery and Neurology*, **5**, 233.

Green, P.W.B. (1977) Anterior cervical fusion. *Journal of Bone and Joint Surgery*, **59B**, 236.

Gregorius, F.K., Estrin, T. and Crandall, P.H. (1976) Cervical spondylotic radiculopathy and myelopathy. *Archives of Neurology*, **33**, 618.

Gregory, C.F. (1964) Complications of anterior spinal fusion. *Journal of Bone and Joint Surgery*, **46B**, 775.

Gupta, A. (1987) Anterior cervical fusions in cervical disc disease. *M. Ch. Orth. Thesis*. University of Liverpool.

Hardin, C.A. (1963) Vertebral artery insufficiency produced by cervical osteophytes. *Archives of Surgery*, **90**, 629.

Hirsch, C., Schajowitz, F. and Galante, J. (1967) Structural changes in the cervical spine. *Acta Scandinavica Orthopaedica*, Suppl. 109.

Holt, E.P. (1964) The fallacy of cervical discography. *Journal of the American Medical Association*, **118**, 799.

Holt, S. and Yates, P.O. (1966) Cervical spondylosis and nerve root lesions. *Journal of Bone and Joint Surgery*, **48B**, 407.

Hughes, J.T. (1978) *Pathology of the Spinal Cord*, 2nd edn. London, Lloyd-Luke. p. 171.

Hutchinson, F.C. and Yates, P.O. (1956) The cervical portion of the vertebral artery. *Brain*, **79**, 319.

Jeffreys, R.V. (1979) The surgical treatment of cervical spondylotic myelopathy. *Acta Neurochirurgica*, **47**, 293.

Jeffreys, R.V. (1986) The surgical treatment of cervical myelopathy due to spondylosis. *Journal of Neurology, Neurosurgery and Psychiatry*, **49**, 353.

Kahn, E.A. (1947) The dentate ligament in cervical spondylosis. *Journal of Neurosurgery*, **4**, 191.

Kellgren, H.J. (1939) Referred pain from deep somatic structures. *Clinical Science*, **4**, 36.

Kelsey, J.L., Gittens, P.B. and Walter, S.D. (1984) An epidemiological study of acute cervical P.I.D. *Journal of Bone and Joint Surgery*, **66A**, 907.

Kikuchi, S., McNab, I. and Moreau, P. (1981) Localisation of the symptomatic level of cervical disc degeneration. *Journal of Bone and Joint Surgery*, **63B**, 273.

King, R.J. and Bonney, G. (1983) Analysis of 82 thoracic outlet explorations. *Journal of Bone and Joint Surgery*, **65B**, 218.

Klein, R.A., Snyder, R.A. and Schwartz, H.J. (1976) Lateral medullary syndrome in a child. *Journal of the American Medical Association*, **253**, 940.

Kobayashi, S. (1974) Tract pain syndrome. *Hawaii Medical Journal*, **33**, 376.

Lane, W.A. (1886) Some points of the pathology of changes produced by pressure in the bony skeleton. *Guys Hospital Reports*, **43**, 321.

McEwan, A.J. (1967) Cervical spondylosis in aetiology of cerebral embolism. *British Journal of Clinical Practice*, **21**, 465.

Mair, W.G.P. and Duckman, R. (1953) False localizing signs in high cervical cord compression. *British Journal of Clinical Practice*, **26**, 215–216.

Martins, A.N. (1976) Anterior cervical discectomy with and without interbody bone graft. *Journal of Neurosurgery*, **44**, 290.

Matsuma, P., Watas, R.L., Adkins, R.H., Rothman, S., Gurbani, N. and Sie, I. (1989) C.T. parameters for the cervical spine. *Journal of Bone and Joint Surgery*, **71A**, 183.

Maurice-Williams, R.S. (1974) Drop attacks from cervical cord compression. *British Journal of Clinical Practice*, **26**, 215.

Murray-Leslie, C.F. and Wright, V. (1976) Carpal tunnel, humeral epicondylitis and cervical spine. *British Medical Journal*, **1**, 1439.

Nagashima, C. (1970) Surgical treatment of vertebral artery insufficiency. *Neurosurgery*, **32**, 512.

Nagashima, C. (1972) Cervical myelopathy due to ossification of posterior longitudinal ligament. *Journal of Neurosurgery*, **37**, 653.

Nakanishi, T., Mannen, T., Toyokura, Y., Sakaguchi, R. and Tsuyama, N. (1974) Symptomatic ossification of posterior longitudinal ligament of cervical spine. *Neurology*, **24**, 1139.

Okawara, S. and Nibbelink, D. (1974) Vertebral artery occlusion following hyperextension and rotation of head. *Stroke*, **5**, 640.

Olssen, Y., Sourander, P. and Kristensen, K. (1972) Neuropathology aspects of root affections in the cervical region. *International Symposium*, **19**, 81–88.

Pallis, C., Jones, A.M. and Spillane, A.D. (1954) Cervical spondylosis, incidence and implications. *Brain*, **77**, 274.

Payne, E.E. and Spillane, A.D. (1957) Cervical myelopathy. *Brain*, **80**, 274.

Phillips, D.G. (1975) Upper limb involvement in cervical spondylosis. *Journal of Neurology, Neurosurgery and Psychiatry*, **38**, 386.

Quast, M. and Liebegott, G. (1975) The pathogenesis of Wallenberg's syndrome. *Bietr. Patholog. Bd.*, **154**, 308.

Riley, L.H. and Richter, C.P. (1975) The electrical skin resistance method in the study of patients with neck and arm pain. *Johns Hopkins Medical Journal*, **137**, 69.

Rogers, L. (1961) The surgical treatment of cervical spondylotic myelopathy. *Journal of Bone and Joint Surgery*, **43B**, 3.

Sager, P. (1972) The accuracy of radiological diagnosis in the cervical spine. *Proceedings of International Symposium on Cervical Pain*, **19**, 49. Oxford, Pergamon Press.

Saunders, J.B. de C.M. and Inman, V.T. (1939) Desiccation and elasticity in the intervertebral disc. *International Abstracts of Surgery*, **69**, 14.

Schneider, E. (1974) Disturbance of sexual function in non traumatic spinal disease. *Fortschrift Neurol-Psychiatrie*, **42**, 562.

Smith, D.R., Vanderark, G.D. and Kempe, L.G. (1971) Cervical spondylosis causing vertebro-basilar insufficiency. *Journal of Neurology, Neurosurgery and Psychiatry*, **34**, 388.

Stuart, D. (1975) Dysphagia due to cervical osteophytes. *Journal of Bone and Joint Surgery*, **57B**, 405.

Stuart, D. (1989) Dysphagia due to cervical osteophytes. *International Orthopaedics*, **13**, 95.

Sullivan, H.G., Harrison, J.W., Vines, F.S. and Becker, D. (1975) Embolic posterior cerebral artery occlusion secondary to spondylotic vertebral artery compression. *Journal of Neurosurgery*, **43**, 618.

Summers, B.N. and Eisenstein, S.M. (1989) Donor site pain from the ilium. *Journal of Bone and Joint Surgery*, **71B**, 677.

Taylor, A.R. and Byrnes, D.P. (1974) Foramen magnum and high cervical cord compression. *Brain*, **97**, 473.

Tchang, S.P.K. (1974) The spino-laminar line. *Journal of the Association of Canadian Radiologists*, **25**, 224.

Tokay, F. and Stachowski, B. (1974) Trauma of cervical vertebral column compounded by vertebral artery insufficiency. *Patologi Polska*, **25**, 445.

Tondbury, G. (1972) The behaviour of the cervical discs during life. *Proceedings of the International Symposium on Cervical Pain*, 59.

Torg, J.S., Pavlov, H., Gennario, S. *et al.* (1986) Neurapraxia of the cervical spinal cord. *Journal of Bone and Joint Surgery*, **68A**, 1355.

Uttley, D. and Monro, P. (1989) Neurosurgery for cervical spondylosis. *British Journal of Hospital Medicine*, **42**, 62.

Verbiest, H. (1968) A lateral approach to the cervical spine. *Journal of Neurosurgery*, **28**, 191.

Wallenberg, A. (1897) Embolie der arterie cerebellaris postero inferior sinistra. *Archiv für Psychologie*, **27**, 504.

Watson-Jones, R. (1932) Spontaneous hyperaemic dislocation of the atlas. *Proceedings of the Royal Society of Medicine*, **25**, 586.

Whitecloud, T.S. III and Seago, R.A. (1987) Cervical discogenic syndrome. *Spine*, **12**, 313.

Wilkinson, M. (1960) The morbid anatomy of cervical spondylosis and myelopathy. *Brain*, **83**, 489–617.

Williams, R.W. (1983) Microsurgical foraminotomy. *Spine*, **8**, 708.

Yoss, R.E., Corbin, K.B., MacCurdy, C.S. and Love, J.G. (1957) Significance of symptoms and signs in localization of involved root in cervical disc prolapse. *Neurology*, **7**, 673.

8 The cervical spine in rheumatic disease

'For Rheumatism or Stiffness
Make an ointment with butter, rue, Frankincense and
three pennyworth of the Blessed Water. Anoint three
times per week for a Summer's month.'
Of the medical practice of the celebrated Rhiwallon and
his sons, of Myddfai. Thirteenth Century. Translated
from the Welsh in 1861 by John Pughe FRCS of
Aberdovey.

Radiography will demonstrate subluxation of the cervical spine in an appreciable number of patients suffering from rheumatoid arthritis, but even with gross radiographic change, neurological damage can be minor or even absent (Smith, Benn and Sharp, 1972; Pellicci *et al.*, 1981). The tendency to natural resolution of subluxation is strong and neurological deterioration uncommon (Mathews, 1974). Cervical subluxations in themselves do not significantly shorten life in patients with rheumatoid arthritis. The incidence of neurological damage in subluxed spines is low; of 130 patients followed by Smith, Benn and Sharp (1972) for 10 years, only three developed signs of central nervous damage. Patients with cervical myelopathy caused by rheumatoid arthritis have severe, progressive rheumatoid disease elsewhere, in the form of severe peripheral joint disease and also as extra-articular manifestation, particularly interstitial lung disease (Saway *et al.*, 1989). These patients die of causes other than neurological damage, although cerebrovascular catastrophe from vertebrobasilar ischaemia in the rheumatoid spine may be more common than is appreciated (Jones and Kaufmann, 1976).

Operations on the rheumatoid cervical spine are dangerous. The patient is a poor surgical risk, approached with a trepidation which does not diminish with experience.

Morbid anatomy

Rheumatoid arthritis is a disease of connective tissue and the pathological lesion in the neck is the same as it is in other parts of the body. The earliest changes are found in the synovium of the 14 apophyseal joints of the cervical spine, and the bursae surrounding the odontoid process. Histological changes in synovium can exist before there are any radiographic signs of joint erosion (Sharp, Purser and Lawrence, 1958). Other tissues affected are the intervertebral discs and extradural alveolar connective tissue. Rheumatoid granulation tissue has been found in the bone marrow spaces of vertebral bodies. This granulation tissue then invades and destroys the disc (Gibson, 1957). Synovitis is followed by juxta-articular erosion. The capsular ligaments, and the restraining ligaments of the odontoid, are stretched or destroyed (Hotta *et al.*, 1989). Subluxation occurs, most frequently at the atlanto-axial levels but also in the lower cervical spine (Ferlic *et al.*, 1975). The extradural spaces are occupied by rheumatoid granulation tissue and sequestrated disc material, and subluxation may be as much due to adaptive change as it is to instability. Ankylosis occurs at the subluxed segments as the disease burns itself out.

Atlanto-axial subluxation can only occur if the alar and apical ligaments of the odontoid have been stretched or destroyed by granulation tissue, or if the odontoid has been eroded to the point of fracture. The blood supply of the odontoid is such that avascular necrosis may follow erosion (see Chapter 3). The process may disappear completely. The forward displacement of the atlas on the axis may become fixed by rheumatoid tissue between the odontoid and the anterior arch of the atlas. If the odontoid is fractured by erosion the tip may come to lie between the alar ligament and the cord. Posterior displacement of the atlas is sometimes seen.

Progressive disease at the atlanto-axial joints will allow upward migration of the odontoid into the foramen magnum where it may indent and deform the cord. Such upward migration is only seen in patients with severe generalized rheumatoid arthritis.

Diagnostic imaging of the rheumatoid cervical spine

The changes thus described can be demonstrated by standard radiography. Lateral films in flexion and extension will demonstrate any instability, or, equally important, any fixed displacement. If management is to be conservative, these films will suffice. The improved detail of contrast myelography, computed tomography and magnetic resonance imaging is necessary if operative intervention is planned.

Standard radiography

The early radiographic changes are those of rheumatoid arthritis in general. Decreases in bone density and juxta-articular erosions reflect hyperaemia and the growth of granulation tissue. These appearances are first seen at the apophyseal joints of the upper cervical spine; vertebral body erosion and narrowing of disc spaces follow and spread to the lower spine. There is a relative absence of end plate sclerosis and osteophyte formation unless the rheumatoid disease attacks a spine already showing signs of degenerative spondylosis.

In the later stages, subluxation of cervical vertebrae will be seen. It may be possible to demonstrate reduction of this subluxation but, in time, the displacement becomes fixed and irreducible as ankylosis occurs.

Forward displacement of the atlas on the axis is assessed by measuring the distance between the anterior arch of the atlas and the odontoid. In the adult the gap should not exceed 5 mm.

Rostral migration of the odontoid is assessed by measuring the position of the axis relative to the foramen magnum. This can be

difficult. Various lines and measurements have been described. McGregor's line is the most useful (Figure 8.1). It is drawn between the posterior edge of the hard palate and the lowest prominence of the occiput. It runs between two fixed points and is constant, but the vertical height of the occiput above the arch of the atlas varies as the head is flexed or extended. The tip of the odontoid should not protrude more than 5 mm above this line (McGregor, 1948). It may not be possible to draw McGregor's line because of problems in identifying the hard palate (Kawaida, Sakou and Morizono, 1989). Another method relates the sagittal diameter of the atlas to the odontoid. The sagittal diameter is measured between the centres of the anterior and posterior arches of the atlas (Figure 8.2). The vertical line of the odontoid is projected upwards from the sclerotic ring of the body of the axis until it intersects the first line. This measurement should be at least 13 mm (Ranawat *et al.*, 1979).

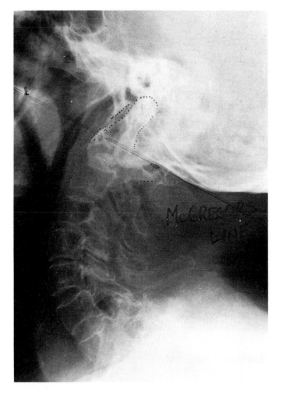

Figure 8.1. McGregor's line.

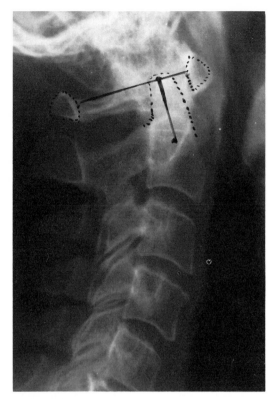

Figure 8.2. Ranawat's line.

Atlanto-axial subluxation can appear early in the progress of rheumatoid cervical disease; upward migration of the odontoid is a sign of late disease and is of poor prognostic import. As the upward migration progresses there will be an apparent improvement of the forward subluxation as the atlas beds down on the odontoid.

Subaxial subluxation can occur at one or more levels, producing the characteristic 'stepladder' picture. In early disease, lateral films in flexion and extension will demonstrate instability with the subluxation reducing in extension (Park, O'Neil and McCall, 1979). In later disease, and almost invariably when clinical signs of myelopathy are present, the subluxation has become irreducible. If flexion and extension myelographic films are then examined it will be seen that movement occurs, not at the subluxed segments, but at the junctional levels between subluxation and normal alignment – and that the dye column is compressed at these levels in extension.

Computed axial tomography

Sagittal and three dimensional reconstruction of CT scanning can demonstrate relationships at the craniocervical junction with greater clarity than standard radiography. Dynamic studies of the flexed and extended spine will show intermittent pressure effects of bone and rheumatoid granulation tissue on the brain-stem and cord (Stevens, Kendall and Crockard, 1986).

Magnetic resonance imaging

The newer methods of imaging, magnetic resonance imaging even more than computed tomography, give detailed information about the spatial relationship of bone and soft tissue in the upper cervical canal. Evaluation of patients with myelopathy using MRI has confirmed that pannus around the atlanto-axial 'joint', and around the odontoid can cause significant cord compression (Longley, Quisling and Sypert, 1987). The clinical assessment of neurological defects in patients with severe rheumatoid arthritis is difficult because of peripheral joint disease. It is becoming possible to make that assessment by imaging, and to recommend operative interference if there is significant diminution of canal capacity (Dvorak *et al.*, 1989).

CT and MRI are expensive; MRI is three times as expensive as CT and it has been estimated that at least 12 scans a day are necessary to meet costs (Hill, 1986; Sinclair, 1988). In the management of rheumatoid myelopathy it is not necessary to have both. The wide availability of CT means that it will remain the first line investigation in most centres for the foreseeable future.

The natural history of rheumatoid arthritis

It is shared experience, and well documented, that rheumatoid involvement of the cervical spine is common and benign. The presence of radiographic abnormality alone, in the absence of neurological signs, does not adversely affect survival. The radiological signs tend to increase in severity with the passage of time but this change is not accompanied by a parallel increase in neurological damage. Pain from rheumatoid neck disease tends to improve in time. Neurological deterioration, and the development of intractable pain, are associated with the progress of severe peripheral joint disease and extra-articular rheumatoid such as vasculitis, cardiomyopathy and interstitial lung disease (Smith, Benn and Sharp, 1972; Mathews, 1974; Nakano, 1975; Pellicci *et al.*, 1981; Rana, 1989). Cervical involvement may not occur until perhaps 25 years into the disease; and sudden deterioration of myelopathy, and peripheral disease may occur after a period of apparent stability. Detection of neurological deterioration is difficult in these severely disabled patients and it is fatally easy to misinterpret a progressive neurological lesion as a manifestation of peripheral disease. Meijers *et al.* (1974) have described 'alarm signals' which should alert suspicion:

1 Intractable neck pain radiating to the occiput.
2 Disturbed bladder function.
3 Flaccid weakness in the arms.
4 'Jumping legs' (spinal automatism).
5 Paraesthesia in the fingers and feet.
6 Numbness in the fingers and feet.
7 'Marble sensation' in the limbs and trunk.

Once myelopathy has set in, progressive deterioration is inevitable unless it is arrested by operative interference. Sudden death has been reported in association with atlanto-axial subluxation (Jones and Kaufmann, 1976; Yaszemski and Shepler, 1990), and of course the true incidence of death due to rheumatoid cervical disease can never be known (Webb, Hickman and Brew, 1968).

Management

The benign natural history of this condition dictates that management should be expectant and symptomatic only, in the majority. Severely disabled patients should be carefully observed for any signs of neurological involvement. The indications for operative intervention are clear:

1 Intractable pain. This is referred into the occiput and is evidence of C1/2 and C2/3 disease. It is an indication for occipitocervical fusion.

2 Cervical myelopathy. The alarm signs of Meijers should alert suspicion. Once myelopathy has been diagnosed, operation should be advised. Further deterioration is inevitable and the best results follow early intervention.
3 Radiographic evidence of severe compromise of the canal, or gross atlanto-axial subluxation.

The objectives of operation are to statilize the spine, to decompress the spinal cord if necessary, and to reduce subluxation, if necessary (Heywood, Learmonth and Thomas, 1988a). The first of these objectives is paramount. Rheumatoid granulation tissue will absorb with splintage, and decompression or reduction of subluxation may not be necessary (Jeffreys and Kyd, 1978; Heywood, Learmonth and Thomas, 1988b). Stabilization should be by posterior fusion. Anterior decompression can be performed at a later operation if there is no neurological recovery. A strong case has been made for anterior, if necessary, transoral decompression and posterior fusion to be done as one operative procedure (Brattstrom, Elner and Granholm, 1973; Crockard, Pozo and Ransford, 1986; Ransford, 1987).

These patients are poor anaesthetic risks. In addition to their severe peripheral disease, and neurological problems, they may have cardiovascular or pulmonary problems. They are elderly, usually on steroids and have poor resistance to wound infection. The morbidity and mortality figures make depressing reading (Hopkins, 1967; Crellin, MacCabe and Hamilton, 1970; Ranawat *et al.*, 1979; Saway *et al.*, 1989).

Operations on the rheumatoid neck are dangerous. The results are often disappointing. The best results follow early diagnosis of neurological involvement. The newer methods of imaging offer an opportunity to identify early involvement when clinical assessment is well nigh impossible. Such patients will be under the care of a rheumatologist who will be responsible for referring them for operation. Good liaison between rheumatologist and surgeon is vital and our results show the benefit of such cooperation. We have reviewed 388 patients treated over a 24-year period (1964–1986) at Oswestry (unpublished study). Forty-one operations were performed in 38 patients. Of these three received anterior interbody fusion, one was decompressed by laminectomy. The remainder were fused posteriorly, nine by atlanto-axial fusion and 28 by occipitocervical fusion with or without internal fixation (Figures 8.3–8.8).

We obtained neurological improvement in over 75 per cent of our patients, and relief of pain in all. One patient died in the immediate postoperative period, and one some weeks later (Gupta A., Roberts M., Jeffreys T.E., O'Connor B.T., personal communication).

The problems of management of rheumatoid cervical spondylitis are not yet solved. Prognosis remains difficult in the individual; clinical assessment is almost impossible in the elderly disabled patient. Too often the indications for operation only become apparent after irreversible damage has occurred. The correct operative solution is not yet agreed. We have a long way to go.

The cervical spine in ankylosing spondylitis

Individuals who inherit the histocompatability antigen HLA B27 are likely to acquire ankylosing spondylitis (Brewerton, 1976). It is not an uncommon condition and the diagnosis should be suspected in any young man who complains of low back pain which is present on waking in the mornings, or made worse by sitting.

The target tissue in ankylosing spondylitis is the junctional area between articular cartilage and subchondral bone. Cartilage is eroded by invasion from below, in distinction from the creeping surface erosion of rheumatoid pannus (Gibson, 1957). This destruction of cartilage explains the tendency to bony ankylosis of synovial joints but does not explain the ossification of periarticular structures such as the longitudinal ligaments of the spine.

The natural history of ankylosing spondylitis is, on the whole, benign. Even in those few patients who progress to total spinal rigidity, sound medical treatment, and aggressive physiotherapy, should prevent the end result of gross kyphosis.

Early diagnosis depends on a high level of suspicion. Thorough clinical examination will reveal early segmental rigidity of the spine, and decreased chest expansion as a result of

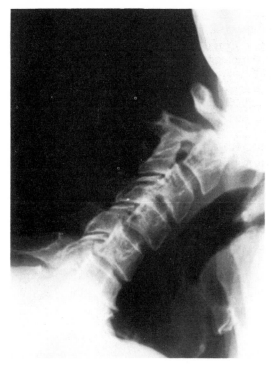

Figure 8.3. Atlanto-axial subluxation in rheumatoid arthritis.

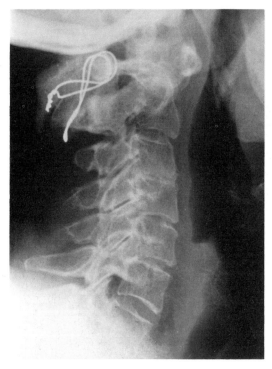

Figure 8.4. Posterior atlanto-axial fusion with autogenous iliac bone graft (Gallie type fusion).

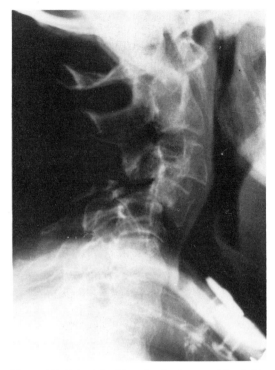

Figure 8.5. Subaxial subluxation in rheumatoid arthritis.

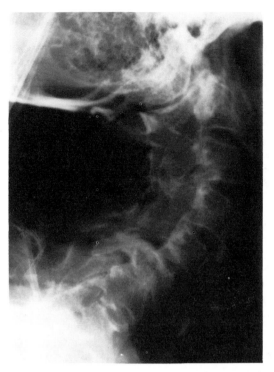

Figure 8.7. Combined atlanto-axial and subaxial subluxation in rheumatoid arthritis.

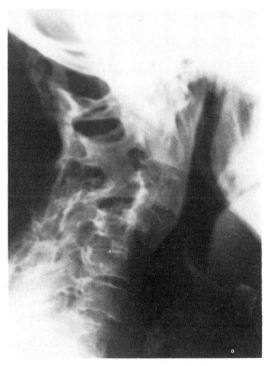

Figure 8.6. Long posterior fusion in situ.

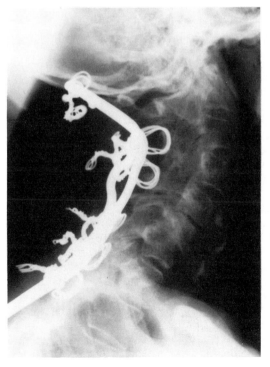

Figure 8.8. Occipitocervical fusion with internal fixation (Ransford loop).

costovertebral disease (Ebringer *et al.*, 1978). Early radiological changes include sacroiliac erosions, and 'squaring' of lumbar vertebral bodies. All patients with iritis or anterior uveitis, and all patients with Crohn's disease or ulcerative colitis should be investigated for ankylosing spondylitis.

When the disease affects the neck it is florid. The degree of ankylosis varies from involvement of two or three lower cervical segments to total neck fusion. Lateral flexion, reflecting lower segment involvement, is the first movement to be restricted, despite the classic picture of increasing flexion deformity (O'Driscoll, Jayson and Baddeley, 1978).

Management of the disease is medical. Nonsteroidal anti-inflammatory drugs are effective in controlling pain. Radiotherapy, once popular and still recognized as effective in relieving symptoms, and possibly arresting progress, has been discontinued because of the risks of post-irradiation leukaemia. Physical treatment is directed towards maintaining an erect posture, remembering that disease of the hip joints can produce flexion deformity even if the back and neck are straight.

Problems arise in the cervical spine with three complications of the late disease.

1 Atlanto-axial subluxation.
2 Hyperextension injury to an ankylosed cervical spine.
3 Flexion deformity of the cervical spine.

Atlanto-axial subluxation (AAS)

The incidence of this complication is variously reported. The old confusion between rheumatoid spondylitis and ankylosing spondylitis produced exaggerated figures. It must be a very rare occurrence overall in the disease. It occurs when active disease in the atlanto-axial articulation develops in the presence of a stiff lower cervical spine. As always in AAS, considerable displacement can occur before neurological signs appear. The absence of peripheral small joint disease facilitates early detection of neurological signs. Unilateral disease will permit collapse of a lateral mass and the patient may present with torticollis.

Radiographic assessment can be difficult. Through mouth radiography may be precluded by temporomandibular ankylosis. CT scanning

is useful in demonstrating rotary subluxation (Leventhal, Maguire and Christian, 1990). Gentle reduction with splintage may allow spontaneous fusion in a good position. The neck must not be allowed to fuse in extension. Occipitocervical fusion has been advocated, but this should not prove necessary.

Hyperextension injury of the cervical spine

The rigidity of the spine in ankylosing spondylitis renders it vulnerable to injury. Unable to extend, the cervical spine readily fractures if a blow is inflicted on the face or head. The fracture is characteristically horizontal, through the level of a fused disc space (Figure 8.9). The fracture may open anteriorly and fall closed again leaving no residual displacement, or the upper segment may be horizontally displaced backward. In

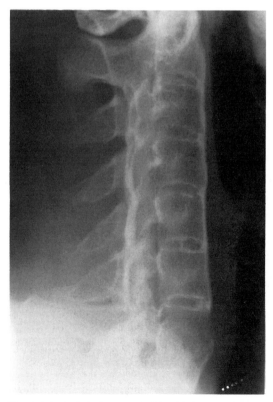

Figure 8.9. Ankylosing spondylitis with fracture through C7. (Mr El Masri's case).

either event the incidence of cord damage is high (Graham and Van Peteghem, 1989; Taylor and Blackwood, 1948). Most fractures occur through the lower cervical spine (Figure 8.10), but cases have been reported at C2, and even through the odontoid (McCall, El Masri and Jaffray, 1985; Kaplan, Tun and Sarkarati, 1990).

A rigid cylinder snapped in half, whether the two ends of the tube are separated or not, is an unstable system. Fractures of the spondylitic neck must be treated with great respect and handled gently. This is particularly important when the patient is transported from the scene of the accident. It must be remembered that in these patients the cervical spine is normally in flexion. Extension of the neck is dangerous. Management of these patients is conservative. Operative treatment is unnecessary and dangerous, having a 50 per cent mortality rate (Burke, 1971; Murray and Persellen, 1981). The neck is stabilized by skull traction. The patient should be transferred to a spinal injuries unit for specialist nursing. After 8 weeks the patient can be mobilized in a well-fitting collar, and union can be expected within 3 months.

Simmons and Duncan (1978) have advanced the hypothesis that the increasing cervical flexion of the severe case is due to wedge fractures of the lower cervical vertebral bodies. Support is lent to this view by a report of three cases of flexion injury, resulting in fractures of the body and facets. The fractures were stable and not associated with cord damage (Simmons and Duncan, 1978; Surin, 1980).

It has been said that if the fracture occurs in a severely deformed spine, and the patient is fortunate enough to escape tetraplegia, the opportunity to achieve an improved position of extension should be seized (Hudson, 1972). This advice is to be accepted cautiously.

Flexion deformity of the cervical spine

Severe flexion deformities result from untreated or inadequately managed disease and are uncommon. The hips and lower spine are more usually the site of deformity. Correction of hip stiffness, and deformity, by total hip replacement is now standard. Most spinal deformity is of the thoracic spine. This is corrected by lumbar spinal osteotomy. If residual flexion of the lower cervical spine still persists after hip arthroplasty and lumbar osteotomy to a degree that the patient cannot look ahead, osteotomy of the cervical spine is indicated.

Cervical osteotomy at the cervicodorsal junction is feasible and rewarding. The osteotomy should not be higher because the

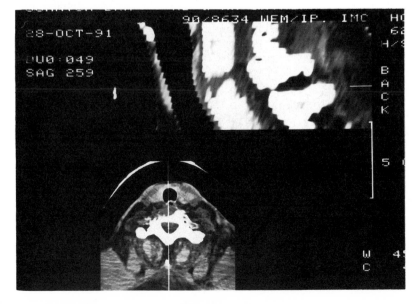

Figure 8.10. CT scan of fracture through C7.

vertebral artery may enter the foramen transversarium at C6, but never at C7. One successful correction at C5/6 has been reported when advantage was taken of a fracture at this level (Hudson, 1972). Simmons advises operating under local anaesthesia with the patient sitting, because intubation or tracheostomy is difficult. The two components of a halo splint are applied before operation and linked together after correction (Simmons, 1969; Simmons, 1977). Armoured intubation may be possible and general anaesthesia by this route is preferable, because if a cardiopulmonary emergency does arise, control is easier to obtain. The operative technique described is essentially that of Smith-Peterson. The cervicodorsal spine is exposed from behind and the dura widely exposed. The osteotomy is through the apophyseal joints, and closed manually with rupture of the anterior ligament and opening up of the disc space. Overcorrection is not advisable. The patient should direct his gaze slightly below the horizontal. The nerve roots at risk are those of C8. The cord must be monitored throughout the procedure and if the signal is lost the spine must be restored to the flexed position (Smith-Peterson, Larson and Andrade, 1945; Law, 1972; Simmons, 1977; McMaster, 1990).

Yeoman (1981) has described a two-stage osteotomy. An anterior osteotomy at C5/6 or C6/7 is done. Two weeks later the dura and emerging nerve roots are extensively exposed from behind and the deformity corrected with minimal force. He advises retrograde intubation via a tracheal puncture if intubation is difficult.

The most gentle procedure has been described by Jaffray. The osteotomy is extended fowards into the body through the pedicles and the wedge is closed on an anterior hinge (Jaffray, personal communication).

Improved anaesthesia and the introduction of halo body splintage has dramatically improved the results of these bold operations. Earlier reports showed a high incidence of complications, but recent series have been trouble free (Yeoman, 1981; McMaster, 1990).

Other seronegative spondylarthropothies

Other conditions which present spinal and paraspinal ossification include a group of inflammatory conditions which have many similarities with ankylosing spondylitis. They do not produce any peculiar surgical problems. Their separate identification is of great interest to the rheumatologist and of great importance in the understanding of the immunological basis of rheumatic disease. The well-read surgeon can display his or her erudition in the differential diagnosis of radiography.

They may be of a common genetic type, attacked by a different exogenous agent. In this group we find psoriatric spondylarthropathy, colitic spondylarthropathy and Reiter's disease.

Reiter's disease, with its triad of urethritis, iritis and arthritis, is of interest to those who are curious about the origin of eponymous diseases. Lieutenant Hans Reiter described one case occurring in the German Army in Italy in 1916. His name has become firmly attached to the syndrome, despite his having been pre-empted by Brodie and Astley Cooper nearly a century earlier; except in France where the disease is known as Leroy-Fessinger syndrome after the two French military surgeons who met it on the Western Front. In France, at least, a prophet is not without honour in his own country. Chauvin after all, was a French deputy.

These spondylarthropathies show fluffy new bone formation at vertebral body margins. The 'squaring' of bodies, seen in ankylosing spondylitis, is not a feature. There is a high incidence of AAS (Killibrew, Gold and Skolkoff, 1973). Senile ankylosing hyperostosis, diffuse idiopathic skeletal hyperostosis and ossification of the posterior longitudinal ligament may all be responsible for cervical myelopathy (Arlet *et al.*, 1976; Fujimoto and Ferayama, 1972; Spilberg and Lieberman, 1972).

In the young, anterior ossification between cervical vertebrae is seen in juvenile ankylosing spondylitis. In seronegative chronic juvenile arthritis there can be interbody fusion (Ansell, 1978).

References

Ansell, B.M. (1978) Chronic arthritis in childhood. *Annals of the Rheumatic Diseases*, **37**, 107.

Arlet, J., Pujol, M., Buc, A., Geraud, G., Gayrard, G. and Latorzeff, S. (1976) Role of vertebral hyperostosis in cervical myelopathy. *Revue de Rheumatisme*, **43**, 167.

Brattstrom, H., Elner, A. and Granholm, L. (1973) *Annals of the Rheumatic Diseases*, **32**, 587.

Brewerton, D.A. (1976) HLA-B27 and the inheritance of susceptibility to rheumatic diseases. *Arthritis and Rheumatism*, **19**, 656.

Burke, D.C. (1971) Hyperextension injuries of the spine. *Journal of Bone and Joint Surgery*, **53B**, 3.

Crellin, R.O., MacCabe, J.J. and Hamilton, E.B.D. (1970) Severe subluxation of the cervical spine in rheumatoid arthritis. *Journal of Bone and Joint Surgery*, **52B**, 244.

Crockard, H.A., Pozo, J.L. and Ransford, A.O. (1986) Transoral decompression and posterior fusion for rheumatoid A.A.S. *Journal of Bone and Joint Surgery*, **68B**, 350.

Dvorak, J., Grob, D., Baumgartner, H., Gschwend, N., Graver, W. and Larsson, S. (1989) Functional evaluation by M.R.I. in rheumatoid arthritis and instability of upper cervical spine. *Spine*, **14**, 1057.

Ebringer, R.W., Cawdell, D.R., Cowling, P. and Ebringer, I. (1978) Sequential studies in ankylosing spondylitis. *Annals of the Rheumatic Diseases*, **37**, 146.

Ferlic, D.C., Clayton, M.L., Leidhott, J.D. and Gamble, W.E. (1975) Symptomatic unstable cervical spine in rheumatoid arthritis. *Journal of Bone and Joint Surgery*, **57A**, 349.

Forestier, J. and Rotes-Querol, J. (1950) Senile ankylosing hyperostosis of spine. *Annals of the Rheumatic Diseases*, **9**, 321.

Fratis, P., Sautarirta, S., Sandelin, J. and Kronttinen, Y.T. (1989) Cranial subluxation of odontoid in rheumatoid arthritis. *Journal of Bone and Joint Surgery*, **71A**, 189.

Fujimoto, K. and Ferayama, K. (1972) Ossification posterior longitudinal ligament of spine. *Proceedings of the XIIth S.I.C.O.T.*, Amsterdam, Excerpta Medica.

Gibson, H.J. (1957) Destruction of intervertebral disc by granulation tissue. *Journal of the Faculty of Radiology*, **8**, 193.

Graham, B. and Van Petegham, P.K. (1989) Fractures of the spine in ankylosing spondylitis. *Spine*, **14**, 803.

Heywood, A.W.B., Learmonth, I.D. and Thomas, M. (1988a) Cervical spine instability in rheumatoid arthritis. *Journal of Bone and Joint Surgery*, **70B**, 702.

Heywood, A.W.B., Learmonth, I.D. and Thomas, M. (1988b) Internal fixation for occipito-cervical fusion. *Journal of Bone and Joint Surgery*, **70B**, 708.

Hill, D.W. (1986) Making N.M.R. cost effective. *British Journal of Hospital Medicine*, **36**, 325.

Hopkins, J.S. (1967) Lower cervical rheumatoid subluxation with tetraplegia. *Journal of Bone and Joint Surgery*, **49B**, 46.

Hotta, Y., Katch, H., Watanabe, J., Azuma, H. and Tauzuki, N. (1989) Non osseous dural compression in rheumatoid atlanto-axial subluxation. *Spine*, **14**, 236.

Hudson, C.P. (1972) Cervical osteotomy for severe flexion in ankylosing spondylitis. *Journal of Bone and Joint Surgery*, **54B**, 202.

Jeffreys, T.E. and Kyd, R. (1978) Cervical spine fusion in rheumatoid arthritis. *2nd International Symposium on Rheumatology*.

Jones, M.W. and Kaufmann, J.C.E. (1976) Vertebro-basilar artery insufficiency in rheumatoid atlanto-axial subluxation. *Journal of Neurology, Neurosurgery and Psychiatry*, **39**, 122.

Kaplan, S.L., Tun, C.G. and Sarkarati, M. (1990) Odontoid fracture complicating ankylosing spondylitis. *Spine*, **15**, 607.

Kawaida, H., Sakou, T. and Morizono, Y. (1989) Vertical settling in rheumatoid arthritis. *Clinical Orthopaedics*, **239**, 128.

Killebrew, K., Gold, R.H. and Skolkoff, S.D. (1973) Psoriatric spondylitis. *Radiology*, **108**, 9.

Law, W.A. (1972) Spinal surgery in ankylosing spondylitis. *Proceedings of the XII S.I.C.O.T.*, Amsterdam, Excerpta Medica, 654.

Leventhal, M.R., Maguire, J.K. and Christian, C.A. (1990) Atlanto-axial rotary subluxation in ankylosing spondylitis. *Spine*, **15**, 1374.

Longley, S., Quisling, R.G. and Sypert, G.W. (1987) Neurological lesions in rheumatoid arthritis. *Arthritis and Rheumatism*, Suppl S92, D1.

McCall, I., El Masri, W. and Jaffray, D. (1985) Hangman's fracture in ankylosing spondylitis. *Injury*, **16**, 483.

McGregor, M. (1948) The signficance of certain measurements of the skull in the diagnosis of basilar impression. *British Journal of Radiology*, **21**, 171.

McMaster, M.J. (1990) There was a crooked man. *The Gold Medal Lecture*, Oswestry.

Mathews, J.A. (1974) Atlanto-axial subluxations in rheumatoid arthritis. *Annals of the Rheumatic Diseases*, **33**, 526.

Meijers, K.A.E., Van Beusehom, B.T., Lyendjik, W. and Duijfies, F. (1974) Dislocations of the cervical spine with cord compression in rheumatoid arthritis. *Journal of Bone and Joint Surgery*, **56B**, 668.

Murray, A.C. and Persellen, R.H. (1981) Cervical fracture complicating ankylosing spondylitis. *American Journal of Medicine*, **70**, 1033.

Nakano, K.K. (1975) Neurologic complications of rheumatoid arthritis. *Orthopedic Clinics of North America*, **6**, 861.

O'Driscoll, S.L., Jayson, M.I.V. and Baddeley, H. (1978) Neck movements in ankylosing spondylitis. *Annals of the Rheumatic Diseases*, **37**, 64.

Park, W., O'Neil, M. and McCall, I. (1979) The radiology of rheumatoid involvement of the cervical spine. *Skeletal Radiology*, **4**, 1.

Pellicci, P.M., Ranawat, C.S., Tsairis, P. and Bryan, W.J. (1981) A prospective study of the progression of rheumatoid arthritis of the cervical spine. *Journal of Bone and Joint Surgery*, **63A**, 342.

Rana, N.A. (1989) Natural history of atlanto-axial subluxation in rheumatoid arthritis. *Spine*, **14**, 1054.

Ranawat, C.S., O'Leary, P., Pellicci, P.M., Tsairis, P., Marchisello, P. and Dorr, L. (1979) Cervical spine fusion in rheumatoid arthritis. *Journal of Bone and Joint Surgery*, **61A**, 1003.

Ransford, A.O. (1987) The cervical spine in rheumatoid arthritis. *Seminars in Orthopaedics*, **2**, 94.

Saway, P.A., Blackburn, W.D., Halls, J.T. and Alarcon,

G.S. (1989) Clinical characteristics affecting survival in patients with rheumatoid arthritis undergoing cervical spine surgery. *Journal of Rheumatology*, **16**, 890.

Sharp, J., Purser, D.W. and Lawrence, J.S. (1958) Rheumatoid arthritis of the cervical spine in the adult. *Annals of the Rheumatic Diseases*, **17**, 303–313.

Simmons, E.H. (1969) Flexion deformities of the neck and ankylosing spondylitis. *Journal of Bone and Joint Surgery*, **51B**, 193.

Simmons, E.H. (1977) Kyphotic deformity of the spine in ankylosing spondylitis. *Clinical Orthopaedics*, **128**, 65.

Simmons, E.H. and Duncan, C.P. (1978) Fracture of the cervical spine in ankylosing spondylitis. *Clinical Orthopaedics*, **133**, 277.

Sinclair, H.D. (1988) The attraction of magnetic resonance imaging. *British Journal of Rheumatology*, **27**, 68.

Smith, P.H., Benn, R.T. and Sharp, J. (1972) Natural history of rheumatoid cervical luxations. *Annals of the Rheumatic Diseases*, **31**, 431.

Smith-Peterson, M.N., Larson, C.B. and Andrade, O.E. (1945) Osteotomy of the spine in rheumatoid arthritis. *Journal of Bone and Joint Surgery*, **27**, 1.

Spilberg, I. and Lieberman, D.M. (1972) Ankylosing hyperostosis of the cervical spine. *Arthritis and Rheumatism*, **5**, 208.

Stevens, J.M., Kendall, B.E. and Crockard, H.A. (1986) The spinal cord in rheumatoid arthritis with clinical myelopathy. *Journal of Neurology, Neurosurgery and Psychiatry*, **49**, 140.

Surin, V.V. (1980) Fractures of the cervical spine in ankylosing spondylitis. *Acta Orthopaedica Scandinavica*, **51**, 79.

Taylor, A.R. and Blackwood, W. (1948) Paraplegia in hyperextension cervical injuries. *Journal of Bone and Joint Surgery*, **30B**, 245.

Webb, F.W.S., Hickman, J.A. and Brew, D.S.J. (1968) Death from vertebral artery thrombosis in rheumatoid arthritis. *British Medical Journal*, **2**, 537.

Yaszemski, M.J. and Shepler, T.R. (1990) Sudden death from cord compression associated with atlanto-axial subluxation in rheumatoid arthritis. *Spine*, **15**, 338.

Yeoman, P.M. (1981) Two stage osteotomy of cervical spine in ankylosing spondylitis. *Journal of Bone and Joint Surgery*, **63B**, 285.

9 Osteomyelitis of the cervical spine

'So long as the disease is active, deformity from disease in the cervical spine can be wholly effaced.'
                                    Robert Jones, 1892.

When Robert Jones wrote the opinion expressed in the quotation he was referring to tuberculous spondylitis (Figure 9.1). He described the causes as 'tuberculous by infection (common) or by inheritance (rare), inherited syphilis and injury from falls, blows and the lifting of heavy weights. The disease also follows and appears to depend on scarlatina, measles, whooping cough and other infectious diseases; but however it begins, or whatever its specific origin the symptoms presenting and the indications for treatment are practically

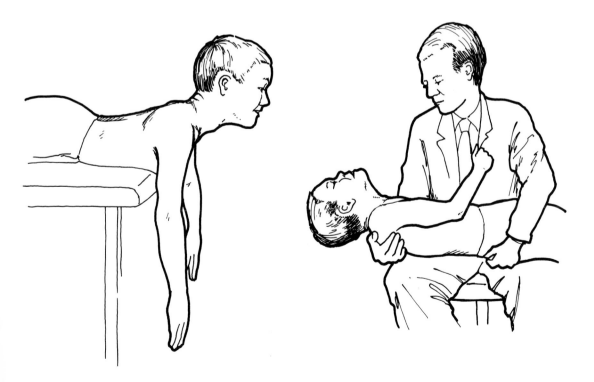

Figure 9.1. Spasm of neck muscles in tuberculous cervical spondylitis (after Jones and Ridlon).

almost identical, and all cases sooner or later show the presence of the tubercle bacilli' (Jones and Ridlon, 1893).

Osteomyelitis of the spine is now recognized as being caused by a variety of organisms. In the western world the infection is due to pyogenic bacteria more often than it is to tuberculosis, although skeletal tuberculosis remains a probability in large cities (Halsey, Reeback and Barnes, 1982; Newton, Sharp and Barnes, 1982; Hodgson and Ormerod, 1990). In the developing world tuberculosis remains an endemic scourge. Whatever the pathogen, there are routes of invasion, initial foci of infection and host/invader reactions that are common to all. Certain groups of people are vulnerable; children and the elderly, the poor and the underfed. Ethnic groups vary in their resistance to disease. The prognosis for skeletal tuberculosis in Indian immigrants is better than it is in the native patients, but this may be due to earlier diagnosis in the immigrants thanks to a higher level of suspicion in the examining doctors (Halsey, Reeback and Barnes, 1982). All forms of spondylitis can present a similar clinical picture; the radiographic appearances can be atypical and are frequently misinterpreted and often the diagnosis is not made until an organism is isolated.

The cervical spine is less often attacked by infection than other regions of the spine. This relative immunity occurs in tuberculous and non-tuberculous infections (Kirkaldy Willis and Thomas, 1965; Griffiths and Jones, 1971; Lifesco, Weaver and Harder, 1985; Emery, Chan and Woodward, 1989).

Direct extension from the nasopharynx or via an open wound is rare. In most cases the lesion is secondary or tertiary to a focus elsewhere. The primary or secondary lesion may be in the lungs, alimentary or genitourinary tract. The skeletal lesion is embolic, the route being the nutrient arteries of the vertebral bodies (Wiley and Trueta, 1959).

Pathology

The onset of vertebral osteomyelitis may be very acute in young children, but is more gradual in adults (Pritchard and Robinson, 1961). The focus of infection is usually in one or two adjacent vertebral bodies close to the annular epiphysis or the vertebral end plate. Uncommonly, the initial focus is in the intervertebral disc, which is not totally avascular (Kemp *et al.*, 1973). Bone destruction follows but the disc may remain as a dangerous sequestrum. Healing by bony intervertebral fusion with minimal kyphosis is the expected result.

In brucellar spondylitis the vertebral bodies are again affected. The disc is replaced by granulation tissue, which extends in front of the vertebral bodies. Reactive new bone forms in this area.

Tuberculous spondylitis, first described by Percival Pott in 1758 and so labelled eponymously ever since, is an osteitis of one or more vertebrae.

The infection may begin in the posterior elements of the vertebrae. When this occurs it is a useful differentiation from pyogenic disease (Digby and Kersley, 1979); but more often than not the lesion is of the vertebral bodies. The tubercles expand and destroy bone. Unlike septic infections, ischaemic sequestra are not formed. New bone formation is not seen in tuberculosis until healing has occurred. The vertebral body collapses, as do adjacent vertebrae, and localized kyphosis follows. The disc may survive after bone has been replaced by caseous material.

Superficial lesions anterior in the body can produce a cold abscess under the anterior longitudinal ligament. Such an abscess, composed of caseous debris, will track under the prevertebral fascia and present laterally. The spinal cord is compressed by abscess material, disc pressure and bony deformity. There is a contributory element of anterior spinal infarction. The dura resists tuberculous infection; the cord is never infected by direct extension.

Diagnosis

Many organisms can cause pyogenic spondylitis, and the literature abounds with reports of cases due to a previously unheard-of pathogen. There are no pathognomonic signs of individual infection and a precise diagnosis must await the isolation of the organism. This may never be found and the diagnosis is made on the results of treatment or the natural outcome of the disease.

Clinical features

Cervical spondylitis is rare. It is more common in children and the elderly. There may be a history of injury (Pritchard and Robinson, 1961). Pyogenic spondylitis often follows urinary infection. A history of previous tuberculosis is significant. Reactivation of tuberculous disease after apparent cure, for reasons that are not understood, is seen in immmigrants to the UK (MRC Tuberculosis Survey, 1982).

The presenting symptom is persistent neck pain, unaffected by posture or physical activity. This may be referred into the head or arms. There will be muscle spasm, limited and painful neck movement, perhaps fixed deformity such as torticollis. A febrile episode may precede the onset of pain in pyogenic disease. There will be fever, general malaise, perhaps a history of night sweats and weight loss. There may be neurological signs at first presentation.

In tuberculous cervical spondylitis an abscess may present, usually laterally behind the sternomastoid but occasionally into the pharynx. Sequestra have been spat out (Hilton, 1863).

The severity of the symptoms will depend on the virulence of the infection, the resistance of the patient and the length of the history. The patient may be an extremely ill child. Before the introduction of antibiotics, staphylococcal osteomyelitis of the spine was a lethal affliction (Butler, Blusger and Perry, 1941). The child may have been unwell for some time. In adults the presentation is more often chronic with constant, but not severe, neck pain and vague malaise. Skeletal tuberculosis can present in different ways in different populations in different parts of the world. Indian immigrants to the UK suffering from tuberculosis tend to present more acutely and to have a better prognosis than indigenous patients. In Saudi Arabia, the UK and North America, spinal tuberculosis is seen in adults while in South East Asia and Africa it is a disease of children (Lifesco, Weaver and Harder, 1985).

Neurological defects are not commonly found on first presentation although they should be carefully sought. Frankel's grading of neurological defect is useful in assessing progress (Frankel, Hancock and Hyslop, 1969). Tertiary referral centres will see a higher incidence of neurological defect, and will observe less frequent neurological damage in the upper cervical than in the subaxial spine (Lifesco, Weaver and Harder, 1985). This phenomenon is also seen in neoplastic disease and is due to the greater capacity of the spinal canal at C1/2, allowing more space occupying tissue to accumulate before the cord is compromised.

Laboratory investigations

The plasma viscosity of the blood will be increased and the sedimentation rate raised. The white blood cell count will be raised. A polymorphonuclearcytosis will favour pyogenic infection, a lymphocytosis will suggest tuberculosis, but these findings are non-specific and are of more value in assessing progress than in making the initial diagnosis (Kemp *et al.*, 1973).

A positive blood culture is an extremely valuable finding. Unfortunately, the indiscriminate use of antibiotics has made a positive result a rare bonus. It was found in six of Digby's 30 cases (Digby and Kersley, 1979).

Serological examinations for the various bacterial antibody titres give useful information. A rising titre is strong supportive evidence to incriminate an organism.

The urine, faeces and sputum must be examined for bacteria. Urine cultures were positive in 13 of Digby's patients (Digby and Kersley, 1979) and responsible pyogenic organisms have been identified from alimentary sources as diverse as the parotid gland and the biliary tract (Emery, Chan and Woodward, 1989). The importance of recognizing open pulmonary tuberculosis is obvious.

Radiography

The radiographs will be normal initially in acute osteomyelitis. Decrease of the disc space will be seen some 2–3 weeks after the infection begins, followed by rarefaction of the adjacent vertebral bodies. New bone formation and eventual fusion of the affected vertebrae may not be seen until at least 12–16 weeks later. Tuberculosis affects the posterior elements as well as the body of the vertebra, and is associated with a greater degree of vertebral body collapse. A florid new bone reaction is seen in brucellosis (Glasgow, 1976). Salmonella infections typically demonstrate marked narrowing of the disc space with adjacent end plate sclerosis. Soft tissue swelling between the spine and the pharynx represents abscess formation and can be seen in all infections. *It cannot be too strongly stressed that it is not possible to make a diagnosis on radiographs alone.*

A radiograph will show alteration in the density and shape of bone and the presence of a soft tissue shadow (Figure 9.2). These appearances are caused by loss of bone substance, destruction of bone, new bone formation and the extension of the disease outside the confines of bone (Figure 9.3). They are non-specific and may even be due to a neoplasm, although the involvement of a disc and two adjacent vertebrae strongly suggest an infective lesion (Figure 9.4).

Computed axial tomography (CT)

CT scanning demonstrates the locality and extent of a lesion with greater precision than

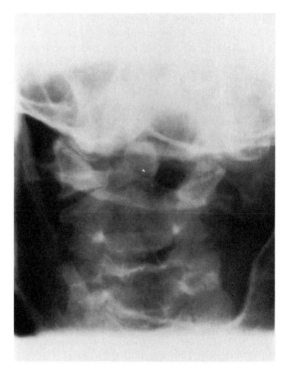

Figure 9.3. Acute osteomyelitis of C1.

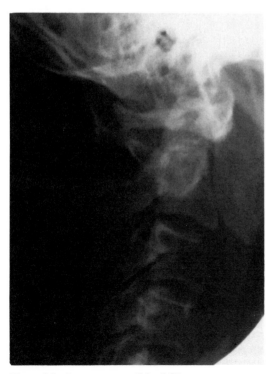

Figure 9.2. Acute osteomyelitis of C1.

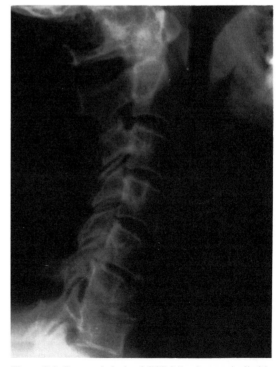

Figure 9.4. Bony ankylosis of C6/7 following septic discitis.

standard radiography. It is of particular value when operative interference is planned.

Magnetic resonance imaging (MRI)

The MRI features of pyogenic spondylitis are peculiar. The T1 weighted images show a confluent decreased signal density at the involved vertebral bodies and intervening discs, while the T2 weighted images show increased signal intensity. The changes are reported to be 'sensitive, specific and accurate' (Bell *et al.*, 1990). Similar appearances are found in tuberculous osteomyelitis. In a tuberculous abscess the calcified areas will not emit a signal and a stippled picture will be seen.

Radionuclide scanning

Isotope scanning reflects bone activity and will therefore detect the hyperaemic changes of inflammation before standard radiography (Majd and Frankel, 1976). It is a non-specific test and as likely to detect neoplastic as infective disease. Gallium-67 is said to be more sensitive to infection than is technetium-99m (Johnson and Jones, 1973).

Isolation of the organism

Access to the cervical body is easy for the aspirating needle and it is a simple matter to obtain tissue for examination (Figure 9.5). Pus may be obtained for smear but it is as well to aspirate tissue for culture and sensitivity assessment, and for histological examination. If antibiotics have been given the aspirate may be sterile. Over 20 separate organisms have been identified as pathogens in pyogenic lesions (Lifesco, 1990). The need to identify the pathogen may be an indication for open biopsy, and all tissue removed at surgical excision must be examined.

Management

Pyogenic osteomyelitis

The diagnosis must be established by biopsy. Closed vertebral biopsy, using the Harlow

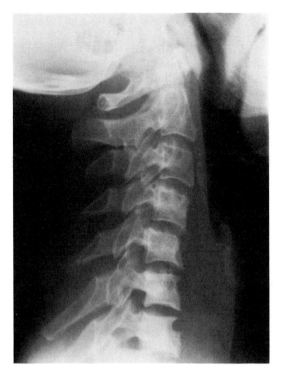

Figure 9.5. Tuberculous osteitis of C7.

Wood needle, should produce enough tissue to establish a diagnosis, but the vulnerability of the spinal cord in the cervical spine is such that conservative management must be critically expectant. In the absence of neurological signs the condition can be managed by splintage of the neck and the administration of the appropriate antibiotic. The response to treatment is monitored by observation of the patient's general condition, the plasma viscosity and white blood count. Radiographic appearances are of less value than the clinical picture in this assessment.

The indications for operative interference are:

1 The appearance of neurological signs.
2 Failure to respond to conservative treatment.
3 Failure to obtain a positive identification of the pathogen by closed biopsy (Emery, Chan and Woodward, 1989).

These indications can be easily interpreted to justify an aggressive surgical approach to all septic lesions of the spine (Lifesco, 1990). Such justification has particular force in the cervical spine, where the consequences of cord damage are profound.

Primary pyogenic lesions of the intervertebral disc in the subaxial spine are associated with a high incidence of neurological damage (Kemp *et al.*, 1973). The only case of pyogenic infection of a cervical disc seen by the author followed provocative discography, and resolved with conservative treatment.

The operative approach should be anterior, as described in Chapter 11. All diseased and sequestrated bone and disc material is removed. If neurological signs are present the spinal cord must be decompressed. The dura is exposed, removing healthy bone if necessary, and cleared until normal dural pulsation is seen. The defect is bridged by autogenous iliac bone as a solid corticocancellous block, extending from healthy bone above to healthy bone below and dovetailed into position so that it is inherently stable. After operation the neck is protected by a halo splint until the graft consolidates.

Brucellar spondylitis

The majority of cases of brucellar osteomyelitis affect the spine, and lesions of the cervical spine have been reported (Lowbeer, 1948; Glasgow, 1976). The diagnosis is usually established only on identification of the organism as the disease is chronic and easily confused with tuberculosis. Management is conservative, using the appropriate antibiotic.

Tuberculous spondylitis

The history of the management of spinal tuberculosis is the history of orthopaedic surgery itself. Many of our orthopaedic centres of excellence began their existence as open-air hospitals for the treatment of skeletal tuberculosis. The treatment of Pott's disease of the spine has been transformed by the introduction of effective chemotherapy and by the development of anterior spinal surgery (Hodgson and Stock, 1960). There was some controversy over the virtues of conservative treatment compared with operative decompression (Konstam and Blesovsky, 1962; Medical Research Council Trials, 1973, 1978, 1982), but the arguments in favour of

the operative treatment of cervical spinal tuberculosis are so cogent that it can be affirmed that the condition should be treated conservatively only if the facilities for operative treatment are not available. The operation is performed under a chemotherapeutic umbrella which begins at least 2 weeks before exploration. The following drugs are given as a daily cocktail: izoniazid 300 mg, rifampicin 600 mg, ethambutol 1200 mg, vitamin B 25 mg. The ethambutol is stopped after 3 months, but the other drugs are continued for 12 months after operation (Lifesco, Weaver and Harder, 1985).

The operation is identical to that described for the management of pyogenic spondylitis. After exposure of the dura a probe is passed up and down to ensure no sequestrated fragments are left in front of the cord. When the evacuated cavity is surrounded by healthy bleeding bone, an iliac graft is firmly morticed into place across the defect.

Exposure of the first and second vertebral bodies is through the open mouth as described in Chapter 11.

Postoperative management consists of efficient splinting of the neck until the graft is demonstrated radiographically to be incorporated. This will take all of 3 months, but the use of a halo body splint will allow the patient to leave hospital once the operative wounds are healed.

References

Bell, G.R., Stearns, K.L., Bonutti, P.M. and Boumphrey, F.R. (1990) MRI diagnosis of vertebral osteomyelitis. *Spine*, **15**, 462.

Butler, E.C.B., Blusger, I.N. and Perry, K.M.A. (1941) Staphylococcal osteomyelitis of the spine. *Lancet*, **i**, 480.

Digby, J.M. and Kersley, J.B. (1979) Pyogenic non-tuberculous spinal infections. *Journal of Bone and Joint Surgery*, **61B**, 47.

Emery, S.E., Chan, D.P.K. and Woodward, H.R. (1989) Treatment of pyogenic vertebral osteomyelitis. *Spine*, **14**, 284.

Frankel, H.L., Hancock, D.O. and Hyslop, G. (1969) The value of postural reduction in the management of paraplegia. *Paraplegia*, **9**, 179.

Glasgow, M.M.S. (1976) Brucellosis of the spine. *British Journal of Surgery*, **63**, 283.

Griffiths, H.E.D. and Jones, D.M. (1971) Pyogenic infection of the spine. *Journal of Bone and Joint Surgery*, **53B**, 383.

Halsey, J.P., Reeback, J.S. and Barnes, C.G. (1982) A decade of skeletal tuberculosis. *Annals of the Rheumatic Diseases*, **41**, 7.

Hilton, J. (1863) *Rest and Pain.* Lecture 5: 111. London, G. Bell and Sons Ltd.

Hodgson, A.R. and Stock, F.E. (1960) Anterior spine fusion for the treatment of tuberculosis of the spine. *Journal of Bone and Joint Surgery*, **42A**, 295.

Hodgson, S.P. and Ormerod, L.P. (1990) Ten year experience of bone and joint tuberculosis in Blackburn. *Annals of the Royal College of Surgeons, Edinburgh*, **35**, 258.

Johnson, G.S. and Jones, A.E. (1973) *An Atlas of Gallium 67 Scintigraphy.* New York, Plenum Press.

Jones, R. and Ridlon, R. (1893) *Contributions to Orthopaedic Surgery.* 17. Printed for private circulation.

Kemp, H.B.S., Jackson, J.W., Jeremiah, J.D. and Hall, A.J. (1973) Pyogenic infections occurring primarily in intervertebral discs. *Journal of Bone and Joint Surgery*, **55B**, 698.

Kirkaldy Willis, J. and Thomas, T.G. (1965) Diagnosis and treatment of vertebral infections. *Journal of Bone and Joint Surgery*, **47A**, 87.

Konstam, P.G. and Blesovsky, A. (1962) The ambulant treatment of spinal tuberculosis. *British Journal of Surgery*, **50**, 26.

Lifesco, R.M. (1990) Pyogenic spinal sepsis in adults. *Spine*, **15**, 1265.

Lifesco, R.M., Weaver, P. and Harder, E.H. (1985) Tuberculous spondylitis in adults. *Journal of Bone and Joint Surgery*, **67A**, 1405.

Lowbeer, L. (1948) Brucellotic osteomyelitis of the spinal column in man. *American Journal of Pathology*, **24**, 723.

Majd, M. and Frankel, R.S. (1976) Radionuclide bone scanning in diseases of the spine. *Radiologic Clinics of North America*, **15**, 185.

Medical Research Council Working Party on Tuberculosis of the Spine. (1973) First Report. *Journal of Bone and Joint Surgery*, **55B**, 678.

Medical Research Council Working Party on Tuberculosis of the Spine. (1978) Five year assessment of controlled trials. *Journal of Bone and Joint Surgery*, **60B**, 163.

Medical Research Council Working Party on Tuberculosis of the Spine. (1982) A ten year assessment of controlled trials. *Journal of Bone and Joint Surgery*, **64B**, 393.

Newton, P., Sharp, J. and Barnes, K.L. (1982) Bone and joint tuberculosis in Greater Manchester 1969–1979. *Annals of the Rheumatic Diseases*, **41**, 1.

Pritchard, A.E. and Robinson, M.P. (1961) Staphylococcal infections of the spine. *Lancet*, **ii**, 1165.

Wiley, A.M. and Trueta, J. (1959) The vascular anatomy of the spine and its relationship to pyogenic vertebral osteomyelitis. *Journal of Bone and Joint Surgery*, **41B**, 796.

10 Tumours of the cervical spine

'Loathesome canker lives in sweetest bud.'
Shakespeare. Sonnet XXXV.

Introduction

This chapter discusses tumours arising from, or metastatic to the skeletal elements of the cervical spine. Neural tumours are excluded with the caveat that the presentation of such a tumour may mimic precisely that of a skeletal tumour. Intraspinal tumours can present in orthopaedic clinics and are often not diagnosed (da Roza, 1964; Frazer, Paterson and Simpson, 1977). Neural tumours can produce bony changes by pressure or invasion. The cervical spine may become unstable following extensive laminectomy or anterior decompression (Bailey and Badgley, 1959; Hastings and MacNab, 1968; Shields and Stauffer, 1976).

New growths of the cervical spine present peculiar problems of management. Rapidly growing tumours will produce tetraplegia from direct invasion of the spinal canal, or from subluxation caused by the destruction of bone. Even the most benign and slowly growing tumour, particularly of the arch, will produce tetraplegia if untreated (Madigan, Warrel and McClean, 1974). The proximity of the tumour to the spinal cord can make operative excision, and the achievement of postoperative stability, difficult. Irradiation of a tumour of skeletal or neural origin can cause myelopathy or even malignant change (Sim *et al.*, 1972; Fagelholm, Halka and Anderson, 1974; Dowdle, Winter and Dehner, 1977). Fortunately, new growths of any variety are uncommon in the cervical, compared with the thoracic or lumbar regions of the spine (Bryce and McKissock, 1965;

Dahlin and Coventry, 1967). It is not known why the cervical spine is so spared. Haemodynamic reasons explain the relative infrequency of metastatic lesions. The extensive venous plexuses of the cervical spine drain more into the sinuses at the base of the skull than into the azygos and canal systems; as do the corresponding thoracic and lumbar systems (Batson, 1940; Dommisse, 1974). But even in benign lesions such as aneurysmal bone cysts, the incidence is lower, vertebra for vertebra, in the cervical than in any other part of the spine (Hay, Paterson and Taylor, 1978).

Recent advances in imaging have increased the chances of early diagnosis of cervical spine tumours, and have increased the accuracy of delineation of the growth within the vertebra. Radical surgical excision can be planned efficiently; the increasing use of internal fixation has enhanced the usage of bone grafts in the stabilization of the spine that must follow excision.

Pathology

Tumours of the cervical spine can be classified as primary, either benign or malignant, or secondary.

Primary tumours

Primary extradural bone tumours of the cervical spine are rare, constituting no more than 10

Table 10.1 Primary benign tumours of the cervical spine

Osteoblastoma
Giant cell tumour
Aneurysmal bone cyst
Osteoid osteoma
Simple bone cyst
Osteochondroma
Chondromyxoid fibroma
Eosinophilic granuloma
Haemangioma
Non-ossifying fibroma

Table 10.2 Primary malignant tumours of the cervical spine

Chordoma
Chondrosarcoma
Osteosarcoma
Fibrosarcoma
Giant cell tumour
Plasmacytoma
Histrocytoma

The presentation of these tumours is similar but a precise diagnosis, which can often only be histological, although some tumours have a characteristic radiographic appearance, will assist in prognosis and inform as to the radiosensitivity or otherwise of a particular lesion.

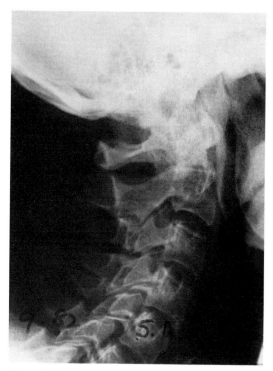

Figure 10.1. Metastasis of C2.

per cent of primary tumours of the axial skeleton (Dreghorn *et al.*, 1990). Reviews suggest that benign and malignant primary tumours occur with equal frequency (Fielding, Pyle and Fietti, 1979; Bohlman *et al.*, 1986). A wide variety of lesions has been reported (Tables 10.1 and 10.2).

Secondary tumours

Metastatic carcinoma is the most common tumour of any found in the cervical spine (Figures 10.1 and 10.2). Other secondary tumours include cervical lesions of haemopoietic tumours such as the leukaemias; and also malignant lesions occurring in previously abnormal tissue such as Paget's disease. Metastases most commonly seen are those from the most common epidermal primary tumours, with carcinoma of the lung heading the list of frequency, followed by breast cancer in women and prostatic cancer in men.

Metastatic deposits in the spine occur in one third of patients dying from carcinoma. Often no primary lesion has been diagnosed in

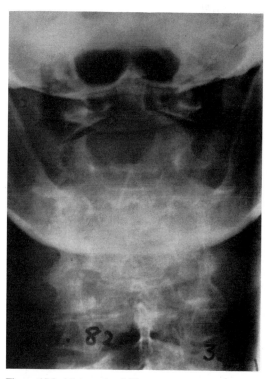

Figure 10.2. Metastasis of C2.

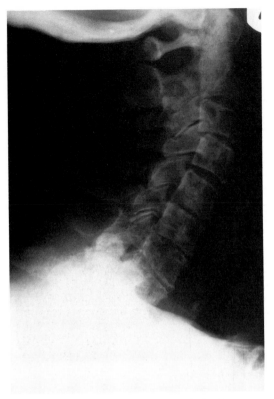

Figure 10.3. Multiple metastases of cervical spine. Primary unknown.

patients who present with cervical metastasis and in an appreciable proportion the primary lesion remains hidden even after the histology of the metastasis has been identified (Figure 10.3) (Shaw, Rose and Paterson, 1980; Wong, Fornaser and MacNab, 1990).

Clinical presentation

Neck pain, or neurological symptoms, in a patient known to have malignant disease elsewhere, will alert the clinician to the presence of a cervical spinal metastasis. Neck symptoms will be the first experienced by the patient if the cervical lesion is primary, and sometimes when it is metastatic. Pain is unremitting and severe. It may be accompanied by muscle spasm and torticollis, particularly in children. There will be local tenderness, possibly a soft tissue mass. Pain

radiating into a cervical or brachial dermatome implies the involvement of a nerve root by the tumour. Signs of a lower motor neurone lesion may follow.

Compression of the spinal cord occurs either by the direct effect of tumour enlargement or by the deformity and instability following destruction of bone. Progress is slow in benign tumours but may be catastrophically rapid in spinal metastasis.

Early signs of cord compression are more likely in subaxial lesions. Tumours of C1 and C2, because of the increased capacity of the spinal canal at that level, can expand to a correspondingly greater degree before compressing the cord. They produce severe neck and occipital pain (Dwyer, Aprill and Bogduk, 1990) and neurological signs may not appear until there has been sufficient bony destruction to produce instability and mechanical compression from subluxation (Phillips and Levine, 1989). If the tumour expands across the foramen magnum the clinical picture can be varied and mixed, with upper and lower motor lesions, nystagmus and ataxia coexisting (Aring, 1974; Taylor and Byrnes, 1974).

Below C2 the cord will be involved earlier. Lateral compression produces the Brown-Sequard syndrome. Sagittal compression produces spastic motor weakness, sensory disturbance and loss of sphincter control in sequence to complete tetraplegia. When the patient is first seen it is useful to classify the neurological defect in degrees of functional severity as described by Frankel, Hancock and Hyslop (1969):

Grade 1   Complete tetraplegia
Grade 2   Some sensation present.
Grade 3   Some motor power but of no practical value.
Grade 4   Useful motor power in arms and hands. Walking with or without aid.
Grade 5   Abnormal reflexes only.

Finally, in the tetraplegic patient, loss of the automatic control of respiration (Ondine's curse) is followed by progressive respiratory failure and death.

The onset of these neurological signs may be insidious or abrupt and their subsequent progress steadily progressive, gradual or staccato.

Investigations

Standard radiography

Standard radiography remains the most generally useful investigation. Some lesions, particularly benign tumours, have characteristic radiographic appearances. Films must be adequate. They must demonstrate all the cervical spine, including through mouth views of C1/2. The craniocervical junction can be difficult to demonstrate because of overlapping shadows. Tomography is obsolete when the newer methods of imaging are available, but still a useful technique when they are not (see Chapter 2).

When the standard films are examined the following changes are sought.

Alignment of the vertebrae

Subluxation, particularly at the atlanto-axial level may follow pathological fracture. Collapse of a vertebral body will result in a kyphos. Paravertebral shadows in soft tissue must be noticed; they are important in the differential diagnosis of abscess or tumour (see Chapter 9).

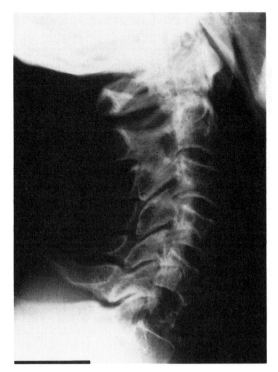

Figure 10.4. Solitary metastasis of C6. Primary breast carcinoma.

Alteration in the shape and size of vertebrae

Benign tumours may expand bone; aneurysmal bone cysts can balloon out into soft tissue. Body, pedicle or lamina can be involved, with posterior elements more commonly affected (Frazer, Paterson and Simpson, 1977). Eosinophilic granulomas cause a characteristic flattening of the vertebral body with 'ghosting'.

Malignant tumours destroy bone. Pedicles disappear, vertebral bodies collapse, fractures occur (Figure 10.4).

Alteration in bone texture

Osteoblastic lesions show increased density of bone on X-ray. Any slow-growing expanding tumour will show sclerosis or scalloping at its margins. Ill-defined areas of increased density suggest prostatic secondaries. New bone formation is seen next to destruction in osteogenic sarcoma. Calcification is seen in osteochondroma and chondrosacoma. Bone destruction implies malignancy. The early changes may be subtle, just the loss of the faint filigree of cancellous bone. Later changes will be clearly visible, perhaps multiple, with fracture, body collapse and dislocation. Disc spaces are not involved in malignant disease, perhaps the only sure distinction from the appearances produced by infection. These general descriptions are not pathognomonic. *No radiological diagnosis can be certain.*

Standard radiography has its limitations. Autopsy has demonstrated occult metastatic spinal lesions not visible on X-ray in 26 per cent of patients with known malignant disease (Wong, Fornaser and MacNab, 1990). Any patient with a history of cancer who presents with unremitting neck pain, must be assumed to have a spinal secondary even if standard films show no abnormality (Harrington, 1981).

Isotope scanning

Technetium scintigraphy has been shown to demonstrate secondary deposits of tumours up to 18 months before the lesion is visible on standard radiographs (Patton and Woolfenden, 1977). The investigation is valuable in demonstrating the presence of multiple, radiographically occult, deposits in the skeleton.

Myelography

Lumbar puncture, and myelography, are dangerous procedures in high cervical tumours. Withdrawal of cerebrospinal fluid allows caudal displacement of tumour and can precipitate catastrophic neurological deterioration. *The investigation should only be performed when there are facilities for immediate surgical intervention.*

Cervical myelography however, either as a standard radiological investigation or an enhancement of computed axial tomography, is a valuable diagnostic tool. Tumours can be differentiated from other space-occupying lesions such as prolapsed intervertebral discs, or syrinx. Tumour margins are outlined; the extent of cord compression is delineated.

Computed axial tomography (CT scanning)

CT is now widely available. It allows sophisticated horizontal imaging of the axial skeleton which, with contrast, allows sagittal or three-dimensional reconstruction. Bone structure, expansion or destruction is demonstrable while the metrizamide outlines soft tissue swelling.

Operations can be planned to approach the anterior, lateral or posterior elements of the vertebra as necessary (Weatherley, Jaffray and O'Brien, 1986; Shapiro, Javid and Putty, 1990).

Magnetic resonance imaging (MRI)

MRI is of less value than contrast enhanced CT in the investigation of bony lesions of the cervical spine. It can provide whole length sagittal images of the cervical column and posterior cranial fossa, with superb demonstration of the neural axis and surrounding soft tissues. It is of particular value in the investigation of lesions at the C1/2 and foramen magnum level.

Haematological studies

The plasma viscosity is higher in malignant disease than in infected lesions. The peripheral blood may be abnormal in haemopoietic tumours.

Biopsy

The indications for operative decompression may be so compelling that histological confirmation of the diagnosis is obtained at the same time as the lesion is excised. If the clinical presentation is less urgent, tissue can be obtained for examination by closed core biopsy, using a 3 mm trephine. This technique provides sufficient soft tissue to permit smear, if a rapid diagnosis is necessary (Findlay, Sandeman and Buxton, 1988). If the need to interfere is less exigent, a definitive diagnosis by a bone pathologist can follow decalcification (Fyfe, Henry and Mulholland, 1983).

Management

The objectives of treatment are to eradicate the tumour, relieve neurological compression and maintain stability of the cervical spine. How these objectives are reached depends on the diagnosis and natural history of the presenting lesion.

Benign tumours

These are rare lesions and their natural history so sufficiently protracted as to allow definitive diagnosis and carefully planned treatment. Some are radiosensitive, but the majority are best managed by excision. Each case must be assessed pragmatically and the operative approach planned to allow complete excision (Bohlman *et al.*, 1986; Weatherley, Jaffray and O'Brien, 1986; Nemoto *et al.*, 1990).

Malignant tumours

Primary malignant tumours of the cervical spine are rare, secondary deposits are common. Metastases may be multiple and the patient terminally ill from advanced malignancy at the time of presentation. An aggressive surgical approach must be softened by common sense. The feasibility of an operation is not an indication for its performance.

Some malignant tumours can be managed conservatively. Prostatic cancers respond to hormone therapy; haemopoietic tumours respond to chemotherapy, some primary lesions are radiosensitive and a painful solitary metastasis without any neurological problems may respond to irradiation. If the diagnosis of a solitary lesion, with no demonstrable primary source, is in doubt, closed vertebral body biopsy using a trephine will give a positive result in 90 per cent of cases (Fyfe, Henry and Mulholland, 1983).

The accepted indications for operative interference are:

1 To establish a diagnosis when closed biopsy has failed.
2 Intractable pain not responding to radiotherapy.
3 Neurological deterioration during radiotherapy.
4 Spinal instability or bony collapse leading to cord compression (Siegal and Siegal, 1989).

These indications may be urgent, the patient presenting as a neurological emergency. Decompression by laminectomy above has given disappointing results. Laminectomy in the presence of vertebral body collapse can be disastrous (Perese, 1958; Bryce and McKissock, 1965; Findlay, 1984). The approach must be to the affected part of the vertebra; anterior or anterolateral if there is vertebral body collapse or destruction of the pedicle, laminectomy if the lesion is in the arch (Raycroft, Hockman and Southwick, 1978; Siegal and Siegal, 1985; Manabe *et al.*, 1989).

Radical excision of tumour and vertebral elements will leave the cervical spine unstable and this instability will negate the benefits of decompression. The spine must be stabilized. Vertebral bodies are replaced by autogenous or allograft bone, and these grafts can be supplemented by internal fixation (Figure 10.5). The use of methylmacrylate is not recommended. It has an adverse effect on the incorporation of bone grafts and has been reported to compress the dura (Dolin, 1989) (Figures 10.6 and 10.7). The available surgical approaches are discussed in Chapter 11.

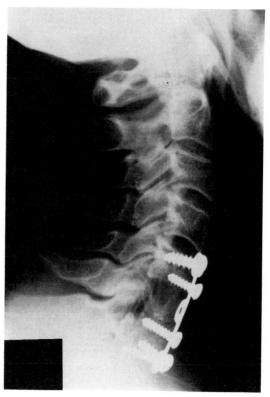

Figure 10.5. Excision of tumour, autogenous bone graft and internal fixation. (Mr C.W. Weatherley's case.)

The prognosis for these patients depends on the tumour cell type, the depth of neurological defect and the site of the lesion. The tumour cell type determines the outcome in each individual. This applies with particular force to primary malignant tumours of bone, which have a dismal prognosis overall. But if an aggressive surgical attack on the lesion in the neck relieves pain, prevents local recurrence and arrests neurological deterioration, it is justifiable. In a series of 15 malignant cervical tumours treated by vertebral body resection and grafting, Fielding and his associates found local recurrence in only two (Fielding, Pyle and Fietti, 1979).

The prognosis for neurological recovery depends on the severity of the lesion when the patient is first seen. Less than 2 per cent of patients with complete cord lesions (Frankel grade 1) show any neurological recovery after decompression of the cord (Nather and Bose,

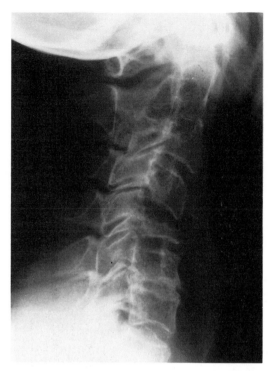

Figure 10.6. Metastasis of C5, with deformity.

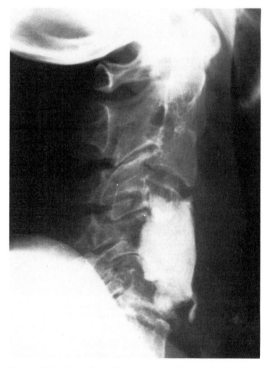

Figure 10.7. Excision of tumour, grafting and methylmacrylate fixation.

1982; Siegal and Siegal, 1989). Early diagnosis not only improves prognosis but may avoid the need for radical operations.

Secondary deposits in the upper cervical spine pose peculiar problems (Phillips and Levine, 1989). The wide sagittal canal at this level allows considerable growth of the tumour before there is compression of the cord. Persistent, severe pain is the presenting symptom. The pain is felt in the neck, and in the back of the head from involvement of the greater occipital nerve (Dwyer, Aprill and Bogduk, 1990). Stability of the upper cervical spine depends on the lateral masses of C1 and C2. Bony destruction can lead to unilateral instability and torticollis. When cord compression does occur it is caused by such instability, with fracture of the odontoid and atlanto-axial subluxation. Diagnosis of these patients is often delayed. Standard radiographs give confusing information and CT scanning is necessary. The prognosis is poor and life expectancy is limited.

Decompression and excision of these lesions is done transorally. The consequent instability requires posterior occipitocervical fusion (Bonney and Williams, 1985; Ransford, Crockard and Pozo, 1986). These procedures, and, it can be held, all cervical cancer surgery, should be carried out in specialized spinal units where surgical, radiological and nursing skills are immediately available. The early diagnosis, and prompt transfer of patients with cervical spine tumours to such centres is the most effective way of achieving the satisfying results that are possible.

References

Aring, C.D. (1974) Lesions about the junction of medulla and spinal cord. *Journal of the American Medical Association*, **229**, 1.

Bailey, R.W. and Badgley, C.E. (1959) Anterior interbody fusion following cervical laminectomy. *Journal of Bone and Joint Surgery*, **41A**, 768.

Batson, O.V. (1940) Function of vertebral veins and their role in the spread of metastases. *Annals of Surgery*, **112**, 1388.

Bohlman, H.H., Sachs, B.L., Carter, J.R., Riley, L. and Robinson, R.A. (1986) Primary neoplasms of the cervical spine. *Journal of Bone and Joint Surgery*, **68A**, 483.

Bonney, G. and Williams, J.P.R. (1985) Transoral approach to the upper cervical spine. *Journal of Bone and Joint Surgery*, **67B**, 691.

Bryce, J. and McKissock, W. (1965) Surgical treatment of malignant extradural tumours. *British Medical Journal*, **1**, 1339.

Dahlin, D.C. and Coventry, M.B. (1967) Osteogenic sarcoma. *Journal of Bone and Joint Surgery*, **49A**, 101.

Da Roza, A.C. (1964) Primary intraspinal tumours, their presentation and diagnosis. *Journal of Bone and Joint Surgery*, **46B**, 8.

Dolin, M.G. (1989) Dural compression secondary to methyl macrylate. *Spine*, **14**, 108.

Dommisse, A.P. (1974) The spinal circulation. In *Scoliosis and Muscle*. (Zorab, P. ed.) London, William Heinemann Ltd. p. 24.

Dowdle, J.A., Winter, R.B. and Dehner, L.P. (1977) Post-irradiation osteosarcoma of cervical spine. *Journal of Bone and Joint Surgery*, **59A**, 969.

Dreghorn, C.R., Newman, R.J., Hardy, G.J. and Dickson, R.A. (1990) Primary tumours of the axial skeleton. *Spine*, **15**, 137.

Dwyer, A., Aprill, C. and Bogduk, N. (1990) Cervical zygapophyseal joint pain patterns I. *Spine*, **15**, 453.

Fagelholm, R., Halka, M. and Anderson, L.C. (1974) Radiation myelopathy of cervical spine simulating intramedullary tumour. *Journal of Neurology, Neurosurgery and Psychiatry*, **37**, 1177.

Fielding, J.W., Pyle, R.W. and Fietti, V.G. (1979) Anterior cervical vertebral body resection and bone grafting for tumours. *Journal of Bone and Joint Surgery*, **61A**, 251.

Findlay, G.F.G. (1984) Adverse effects of the management of malignant spinal cord compression. *Journal of Neurology, Neurosurgery and Psychiatry*, **47**, 761.

Findlay, G., Sandemann, D. and Buxton, P. (1988) The role of needle biopsy in the management of malignant spinal core compression. *British Journal of Neurosurgery*, **2**, 479.

Frankel, H.L., Hancock, D.O. and Hyslop, G. (1969) The value of postural reduction in the management of paraplegia. *Paraplegia*, **9**, 179.

Frazer, R.D., Paterson, D.C. and Simpson, D.A. (1977) Orthopaedic aspects of spinal tumours in childhood. *Journal of Bone and Joint Surgery*, **59B**, 143.

Fyfe, J., Henry, A. and Mulholland, R.C. (1983) Closed vertebral biopsy. *Journal of Bone and Joint Surgery*, **65B**, 140.

Harrington, K.D. (1981) The use of methylmacrylate in the treatment of pathologic fracture-dislocations of the spine. *Journal of Bone and Joint Surgery*, **63A**, 36.

Hastings, D.E. and MacNab, I. (1968) Tumours of the upper cervical spine. *Journal of Bone and Joint Surgery*, **50B**, 436.

Hay, M.C., Paterson, D.C. and Taylor, T.K.F. (1978) Aneurysmal bone cysts of the spine. *Journal of Bone and Joint Surgery*, **60B**, 406.

Madigan, R., Warrel, T. and McClean, E.J. (1974) Cervical cord compression in hereditary multiple exostosis. *Journal of Bone and Joint Surgery*, **56A**, 401.

Manabe, S., Tateishi, A., Abe, M. and Ohno, T. (1989) Surgical treatment of metastatic tumours of the spine. *Spine*, **14**, 41.

Nather, A. and Bose, K. (1982) Decompression of spinal metastases. *Clinical Orthopaedics*, **169**, 103.

Nemoto, O., Moser, R.P., Van Dam, B.E., Aoki, J. and Gilkey, F.W. (1990) Osteoblastoma of the spine. *Spine*, **15**, 1272.

Patton, D.P. and Woolfenden, J.M. (1977) Radionucleid bone scanning in diseases of the spine. *Radiologic Clinics of North America*, **15**, 177.

Perese, D.M. (1958) Therapy of metastatic extradural spinal cord tumours. *Cancer*, **11**, 214.

Phillips, E. and Levine, A.M. (1989) Metastatic lesions of the upper cervical spine. *Spine*, **14**, 1071.

Ransford, A.E., Crockard, H.A. and Pozo, J.L. (1986) Craniocervical instability treated by contoured loop fixation. *Journal of Bone and Joint Surgery*, **68B**, 173.

Raycroft, J.F., Hockman, R.P. and Southwick, W.O. (1978) Metastatic tumours involving cervical vertebrae. *Journal of Bone and Joint Surgery*, **60A**, 763.

Shapiro, S.A., Javid, T. and Putty, T. (1990) Osteochondroma with cervical cord compression. *Spine*, **15**, 600.

Shaw, M., Rose, J. and Paterson, A. (1980) Metastatic extradural malignancy of the spine. *Acta Neurochirurgica*, **52**, 113.

Shields, C.L. and Stauffer, E.S. (1976) Late instability in cervical fractures secondary to laminectomy. *Clinical Orthopaedics*, **119**, 144.

Sim, F.H., Cripps, R.E., Dahlin, D.C. and Ivins, J.L. (1972) Post-radiation sarcoma of bone. *Journal of Bone and Joint Surgery*, **54A**, 1479.

Siegal, T.Z. and Siegal, T. (1985) Vertebral body resection for malignant epidural compression. *Journal of Bone and Joint Surgery*, **67A**, 375.

Siegal, T.Z. and Siegal, T. (1989) Current considerations in the management of malignant spinal cord compression. *Spine*, **14**, 223.

Taylor, A.R. and Byrnes, D.P. (1974) Foramen magnum and high cord compression. *Brain*, **97**, 473.

Weatherley, C.R., Jaffray, D. and O'Brien, J.P. (1986) Radical excision of an osteoblastoma of the cervical spine. *Journal of Bone and Joint Surgery*, **68B**, 325.

Wong, D.A., Fornaser, V.L. and MacNab, I. (1990) Spinal metastases: the obvious, the occult and the imposters. *Spine*, **15**, 1.

11 Surgical approaches to the cervical spine

David Jaffray

'Cursed be the man, the poorest wretch in life,
The crouching vassal to the tyrant wife.'

Robert Burns

Introduction

Operations on the cervical spine ought not to be an everyday experience and they are very unforgiving if you choose the wrong one. Gentle handling is rewarding and a variation in approach is often required. Even specialist spinal centres may not perform cervical procedures in such numbers that permit a vulgar familiarity. I will omit approaches that I consider inappropriate. Occasionally the correct approach to certain cervical problems is only discovered in the anatomy department and cannot be found in any book.

Most cervical operations require a period of preparation. As the skin incision is made the surgeon is bonded to the patient for better or for worse. This is not to suggest that every procedure should be preceded by unnecessary tardiness. If a definite diagnosis has been made then why delay? The real diagnosis may not be the most striking appearance on the X-ray. Blindness to the obvious can tax the most sophisticated minds (Figure 11.1). Generally

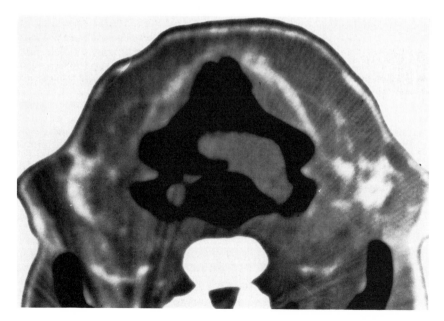

Figure 11.1. Patient complained of torticollis for 5 years. Clinical examination showed brisk reflexes. The skin showed café au lait staining. CT shows a thin crescent of cord at C2. Neurofibromatosis. Two neurosurgeons, one neurologist, one general surgeon and one orthopaedic surgeon failed to make a diagnosis.

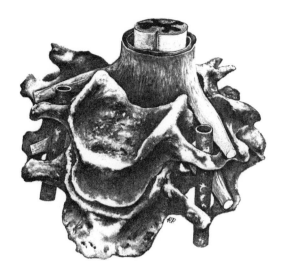

Figure 11.2. Antero-oblique view of vertebral segment.

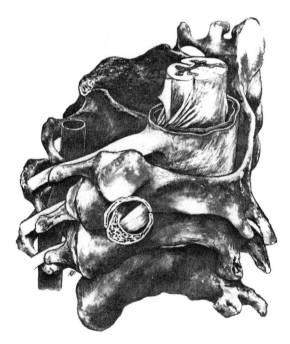

Figure 11.3. Postero-oblique view of vertebral segment with foraminotomy.

can get to know it very well in the anatomy room. Despite its complexity, its anatomy is constant. Surgeons may like to think otherwise and try to make the anatomy fit in with their only surgical approach, usually posterior. This is useless. Define where you want to go. Look at the anatomy. *It* will dictate, not you, the direction of surgical approach.

Do not operate on the wrong level. A good habit is to write the level and side on the patient's relevant arm in the anaesthetic suite prior to the operation with the patient awake. Do not rely on X-rays. They can be incorrectly labelled and I know of a patient explored on the wrong side for a neurofibroma because the CT scan was labelled incorrectly. At a prestigious spinal unit in Europe I was impertinent enough to ask on which side was the patient's radiculopathy. The surgeon had not seen the patient awake. Intraoperative X-rays are imperative but even this can be misleading if the surgeon gets confused at the atlanto-axial junction. Danger can arise if the patient's head is rotated and an oblique film is taken (Figures 11.4, 11.5 and 11.6). An intraoperative X-ray is your legal document that says at least you operated at the correct level. Brief research demonstrated that many surgeons do not share my opinion. What use is a marriage without a certificate?

Operating on the cervical spine should be no different from surgical operations elsewhere in the body. It involves three distinct processes: exposure, preparation and fixation. Each step is important but good exposure, like a good assistant, makes the rest of the operation a pleasure. Never proceed to the next stage before completing the first process. The first two stages, exposure and preparation, are standard, but fixation varies according to the individual preference of the surgeon.

Consent

The patient should know what he faces. There is a risk of paralysis inherent with every cervical procedure. This is more so in a rheumatoid patient. Risks peculiar to the surgery of the cervical spine are damage to the cerebral circulation, and respiratory obstruction. Add the complications of surgery in general, and many patients will have second thoughts. Patients should beware of surgeons who never have complications.

speaking, a healthy preoperative quest for a definitive diagnosis is no bad thing. Do not be tempted into speculative relationships with dubious diagnoses.

The cervical spine may look a simple structure from the outside, but inside it is complex and dangerous (Figures 11.2 and 11.3). You

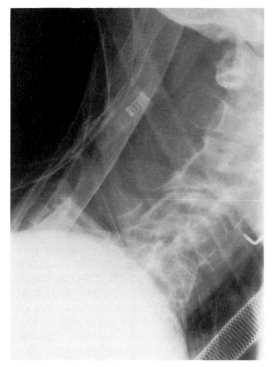

Figure 11.4. First X-ray marker film. I cannot be at C2/3.

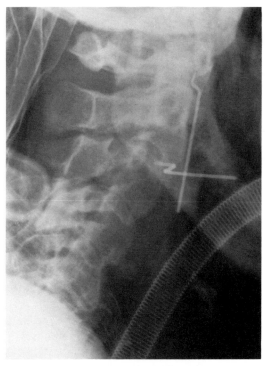

Figure 11.6. A true lateral film. I have been at C2/3 all the time. This X-ray shows how easy it is to reach the odontoid through the anterolateral approach.

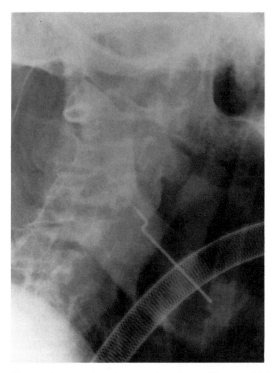

Figure 11.5. Another X-ray marker. I am still not at C2/3.

Anaesthesia

Apart from extensor osteotomies in ankylosing spondylitis, all cervical operations will be performed under general anaesthesia. Occasionally with cases of gross instability an awake intubation is needed. Skill with the fibreoptic laryngoscope is useful.

You may be asked to perform a tracheotomy either electively or urgently. Staff in the postoperative room who are familiar with respiratory obstruction and the use of mini-tracheotomy will save some patients.

Operations at the junctional areas of the cervical spine are uncommon and will be discussed after I have dealt with the mid-cervical spine. The cervical spine can be approached from the front, back or side. Define where you have to go and design your approach accordingly. This may seem to be so basic that you may feel insulted by this suggestion. However, many surgeons, experienced or not, try to use the only approach that they are comfortable with to reach impossible sites. This may be appropriate in surgery elsewhere, but it is not appropriate in the neck. The anatomy of the neck is constant. Unfortunately the neural structures cannot simply be pushed aside as a general surgeon can displace the abdominal viscerae to reach the target site. Look at the cervical skeleton to see if your approach will allow you where you want to go. If not then change your approach. If you cannot, then go no further.

Anterior approach C3/4–C7

Position

The patient lies supine with the head resting on a head rest. I prefer the head to rest on a support rather than on the actual table because it ensures that the neck is uncluttered and allows an image intensifier to be positioned. Traction can be neatly applied using skull tongs or a halo which can be used postoperatively (Figure 11.7). The more conventional halter traction is clumsy and is too near the sterile

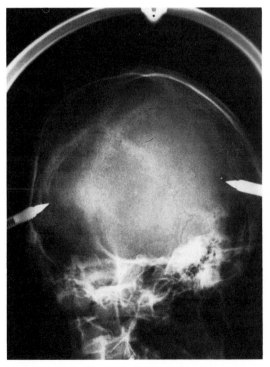

Figure 11.7. Headache for one week. Courtesy of St Elsewhere's. Use skull tongs with care.

surgical field. Drape the patient with care because the middle of a cervical spine operation is not the time or place to be adjusting drapes. Secure the drapes with stay sutures with due respect to skin cosmesis. Have the suction and diathermy safely secured.

Incision

Operate from the side on which you feel comfortable. Too much has been said about risks to the recurrent laryngeal nerve and the thoracic duct which are damaged by clumsiness. There is seldom any gain from a longitudinal incision. A cosmetic transverse incision, particularly if it crosses the midline and is centred on C5, will expose C3–C7. It often helps to separate skin and platysma for a centimetre or two. Divide platysma in the line of the incision. The cleft between sternomastoid and sternohyoid should be apparent. Tease this plane apart ensuring that the carotid sheath displaces laterally with, and under the sternomastoid. The spine and, in particular, the mid-spine between the longus colli muscles should now be both palpable and visible. Find the level by placing a needle in what is thought to be the correct disc space, and take a true lateral X-ray. Bend the needle to prevent it accidentally being displaced into the spinal canal during the manoeuvres to take the X-ray. Now peel the longus colli muscles off the spine using a small periosteal elevator. Prophylactic cauterization of the muscle attachments with the bipolar diathermy prevents unwanted bleeding and keeps the field dry. In due course the cervical spine from C3 to C7 can be exposed. It may be necessary occasionally to ligate the superior thyroid artery. Omohyoid can be easily retracted. The operative field should now be dry. Improve the exposure by placing Cloward type self-retaining retractors under the bellies of the elevated longus colli muscles and another pair longitudinally if necessary. This can be awkward but spend time getting it right. Suture these retractors to the skin. The exposure is now finished.

Posterior exposure occiput–C1

Posterior exposure of the cervical spine is much harder work and more destructive to the tissues than is anterior exposure. Instead of important soft structures that can be swept aside, vascular muscles have to be stripped off the spine. Posterior approaches to the cervical spine are no soft option for surgeon or anaesthetist.

Position

The patient lies prone with the head supported on a frame attached to the operating table. Halo traction can steady the head. Now is a good time to shave off any unwanted hair that strays into the operating field. Infiltration of the operating field with adrenaline is used more often than not. Whether it decreases bleeding is debatable. It certainly can disrupt the normal anatomical planes. If as a result the mid-line is missed, muscle which still bleeds is entered. Surgical drapes do not naturally lie still on the convex surfaces of the skull and shoulders, so secure them now with stay sutures.

Incision

A vertical mid-line incision is used for most procedures. A transverse scar heals quicker and leaves a better scar but it is necessary to check the level with an X-ray. Deepen the incision using a diathermy needle in the mid-line down to the laminae. Sweep the muscles off the laminae using Cobb elevators. When clearing the tissues off the C1 lamina, beware of the vertebral arteries.

The posterior elements crowd together in a space which always seems to be smaller than it should be. Determine the level on a lateral radiograph and while waiting for this, make sure the operative field is dry. The exposure is now complete.

Lateral approach

This is an approach to the vertebral artery. It is seldom used though it can be used to decompress the lateral root canals. More often it is used to approach the lateral masses for tumour resection. The exposure of the lateral elements of C2–4 is the same exposure as the anterior surfaces of C2–4.

Lateral and anterior exposure of C2–4

Position

The patient lies supine on a neurosurgical head rest and is rotated to the opposite side. The incision is an inverted hockey stick cut which begins behind the ear and then runs down along the anterior border of sternomastoid. It is not usually necessary to detach sternomastoid from the mastoid process. Find the accessory nerve a third of the length down the sternomastoid. The nerve is at least the thickness of a pencil lead. The lateral mass of C1 is surprisingly superficial. By gentle dissection find the internal jugular vein and develop the plane behind it. There are no neurovascular structures in this plane so it is vital to enter this space and stay there. The anterior aspect of C2 is now palpable. Slowly develop this plane. Suitably sized and shaped copper retractors placed over the far side of the cervical spine will leave the spine from the base of the odontoid to C4 exposed. The lateral masses are covered by muscle which can now be stripped off the bones.

The lateral masses of C5–7

The standard anterior approach can be used together with strong retraction of the carotid sheath laterally. However, excessive force is undesirable in any cervical procedure so there are two options:

1 Division of the sternomastoid and medial retraction of the carotid sheath.
2 Retain the sternomastoid and mobilize it medially.

The latter is preferable, especially in children.

To excise the lateral masses or to enter the root canals the vertebral artery needs to be freed. This is best done by using a burr to drill through the anterior wall of the canal on to a small right angle probe in the vertebral foramen. The artery can now be lifted out of its canal and either retracted or ligated. The nerve roots above and below lie behind the artery. With these structures suitably protected, the lateral mass can be excised though the posterior half is best removed through a posterior incision. Identification of the nerve roots behind the vertebral artery allows the surgeon to follow them back into the spinal canal.

Junctional areas

Occiput–C2

Odontoid

I believe that excision of the odontoid is the only reasonable operation to be performed on the odontoid. It has become fashionable to fix internally fractures of the odontoid. Not only is this mechanically unsound but the screws themselves occupy more than half the area of bony contact. Type 2 odontoid fractures are uncommon and often harmless. If they have to be stabilized then a simple posterior C1–2 fusion is all that is necessary. The reader is advised not to be tempted into this exercise which has a steep learning curve.

Transoral approach

This is usually a staged procedure. After resection of the odontoid, a posterior fusion is need to hasten the rehabilitation.

Position

The patient lies supine with the head supported on a neurosurgical head rest. Modern retractors (Crockard) have made tracheotomy redundant in most cases. Generous use of adrenalin solutions into the posterior pharyngeal wall makes proceedings dry. The arch of C2 and the odontoid are easily felt. It is best to raise a proximally based rectangular flap of the posterior pharyngeal wall. This flap will not necrose and is easily sutured back at the end of the operation. The margins of the odontoid are obscured by the overlying bursa which can be broken using laser dissection. The arch of C2 and then the base of the odontoid are broken with a burr and the odontoid is removed piecemeal.

For access beyond the foramen magnum it may be necessary to split the hard and soft palate. The service of the maxillofacial surgeon will prevent an iatrogenic cleft palate. Transoral surgery is not often needed even in specialist units. It goes without saying that it can only be contemplated by a few surgeons.

The transoral approach cannot easily visualize the body of C2. The anterolateral approach described earlier is preferable.

Cervicothoracic junction

It is seldom necessary to approach this difficult area. The pathology is often dire and a certain amount of surgical licence is permitted. In theory a sternotomy with limited retraction of the superior mediastinum is feasible, but the access at the end of a long mobile tunnel is not made for precision work. Therefore I advise the approach described by Webb. A thoracotomy through the bed of the second rib after complete division of the muscles along the medial border of the scapula and the erector spinae will expose the target area. Troublesome intercostal neuralgia may be avoided by repair of the intercostal nerve. It can be difficult to identify and preserve the first thoracic root. The damage to the medial parascapular muscles has to be accepted.

Special techniques

Disc excision (anterior)

Disc excision is given a good start by careful dissection with a size 15 scalpel blade and pituitary rongeurs. Distraction of the disc space using Caspar distractors is especially useful. The posterior longitudinal ligament is identified by its fibrous pattern. It is best removed using baby nibblers to create a window, thereby allowing access for the 1 mm Kerosin cutters. Osteophytes arising from the uncovertebral joints can be removed with the kerosin cutters or by forceful upward resection using a 90+ resector. Do not remove the end plates until all manoeuvres at the depth of the disc space have been completed to prevent a sump of blood obscuring the view. It is, of course, up to the individual surgeon to decide if resection of these osteophytes is necessary.

Vertebrectomy

Vertebral body excision is performed for a variety of reasons, including tumour and infection. Exposure has to be of a vertebral body above and below. Disc excision is performed above and below the vertebral body. This indicates the location of the spinal canal. With tumours, sometimes the vertebral body can be simply curetted or even sucked out. More often the vertebral body is hard. An electric burr is then used to drill through to the spinal canal. This is done slowly under irrigation and suction. The back wall of the vertebral body has a different texture and is easily seen. Pass a narrow dissector behind the thin remnant of the vertebral body from above and below. Once the canal has been identified the rest of the excision can be completed without power tools (Figures 11.8, 11.9 and 11.10).

Ligamentum flavum excision–laminotomy/laminectomy

The ligamentum flavum is not a continuous sheet but is split vertically in the midline. This slit is the key to safe resection. Exposure

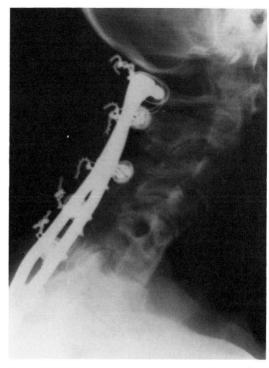

Figure 11.9. The lesion has been excised and the defect grafted.

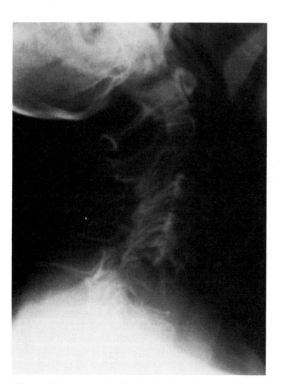

Figure 11.8. A vertebral body has been destroyed by tumour.

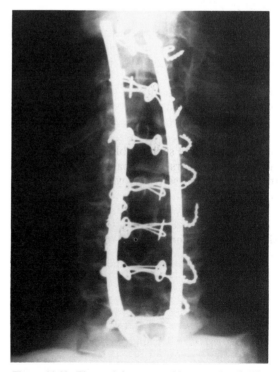

Figure 11.10. The graft is protected by posterior fixation.

requires resection of the overhanging spinous process at its base. The safest way to get through the excess ligamentum flavum is using a bone nibbler, crude as it may appear. Once the slit is identified a Watson Cheyne dissector can delineate the way for the Kerosin. It is now easy to proceed to laminotomy and laminectomy. A high speed burr can be used if the nature of the pathology and the quality of the bone permit.

Foraminotomy

It is imperative to be at the precise level during this procedure and intraoperative radiographic guidance is advisable. A high speed burr can be used to drill through the joint complex. Alternatively, a hemilaminectomy will expose the nerve root which can then be followed laterally. The root lies posterior to the vertebral artery and protects it. It is possible to remove disc prolapses this way but I believe that the anterior approach is preferable.

Bone grafting

Bone grafts must incorporate to achieve fusion. No amount of internal fixation alters this basic fact and legions of failed metallic constructions attest to it. The balance between ironmongery and biology is delicate. (Pathologies like rheumatoid that actively destroy bone do not help.) Fortunately, developments like bone morphogenic protein may help the surgeon overcome such problems. Bone substitutes from cadavers or animals have been tried and failed because they were incompletely denatured. Properly prepared substitutes will return. Glass ceramic materials are here to stay and are ideal for tumour surgery. Meanwhile we continue to use the patient's own tissues.

Preparation of recipient site

Too often this is done hastily towards the end of a stressful operation. Posteriorly there must be a bed of raw bleeding cancellous bone. There are various ways of achieving this. Force is not one of them. A hammer and osteotome have no place in the cervical spine.

Use a low speed high torque burr. Avoid irrigation of bony surfaces. Blood is the best preparation. Anteriorly a graft must have jigsaw precision. The Caspar technique allows distraction of the disc space thereafter compression of the graft. The surfaces of the vertebral bodies should be made parallel using a burr. Do not destroy the end plates beyond bleeding bone or the benefits of distraction will be lost by collapse of cancellous bone. If grafting is needed after discectomy, disc height and cervical lordosis should be maintained.

Occasionally long bone grafts are needed in tumour surgery or for long anterior decompressions. The fibula, if properly countersunk, is effective, despite its obvious design failures. To avoid superficial peroneal nerve damage, take the graft subperiosteally.

Donor sites

Iliac crest

Anterior.

The problems of donor site pain can be so severe that many surgeons have stopped using bone grafts in anterior disc surgery. To minimize these problems grafts must be taken behind the anterior superior iliac spine. Subperiosteal dissection should be the rule. Adequate repair of flaps and a drain are necessary. Repair of defects using ceramics may have a role to play in the future.

Posterior.

Donor site pain from posterior donor sites can be severe. This is because muscles are stripped off the posterior iliac crest and the removal of slabs of cortical bone leaves a raw area which never returns to normal. There is evidence that cortical bone is of little use unless it is used as a strut. The bone forming cells lie in cancellous bone. To avoid donor problems and to use cancellous bone only I advise the following technique. The posterior superior iliac spine and adjacent 10 cm of iliac crest are exposed. An enormous amount of pure cancellous bone can be shelled out from between the intact leaves of the iliac crest. Insert the fresh cancellous bone immediately into the neck and compact it down.

Fixation devices

Much is said about the techniques involved in fixation of the cervical spine. Little is said about the biomechanics of such devices, particularly in the rheumatoid spine where the presence of metal is of radiological interest rather than biomechanical benefit. Anterior plating must surely be sound mechanically on a tension band surface. It is of no use in a rheumatoid spine. The most tried system is that of Caspar. The technique is not difficult but requires a steady hand and generous radiological exposure. A high quality image intensifier is essential if the screws are going to engage the posterior cortex. If the posterior cortex is not engaged with the screws than it is a waste of time using a plate.

Posterior fixation devices are varied. The most common in use is sublaminar wiring. If such wiring techniques are used, short double blunt ended wires (Mehdian) are less likely to pierce the surgeon's hand or the patient's spinal cord. The base of the spinous processes

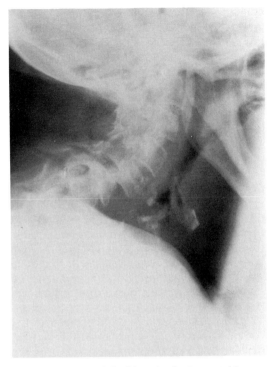

Figure 11.12. Subaxial subluxation in rheumatoid arthritis.

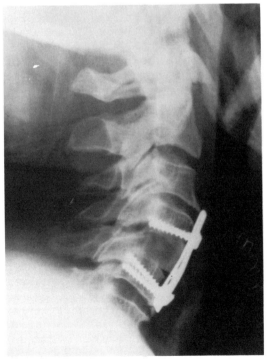

Figure 11.11. The Caspar plate. The screws must perforate the posterior cortex of the vertebral body.

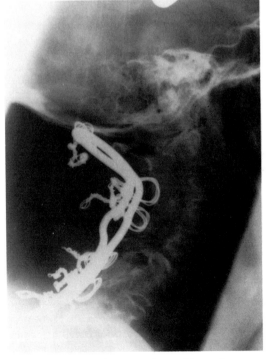

Figure 11.13. Reduction, posterior grafting and occipitocervical fixation.

should not be ignored. If the wires are passed through the true base of the spinous processes a good grip can be achieved. Such techniques have been used for many years to fix reduced dislocations of cervical spines, but their use in a Wisconsin fashion is not to be dismissed (Figures 11.11 and 11.12). Proximal fixation to the skull requires screws through the ridges or combination of burr holes for wires. Use a dental burr for this. The biomechanics remain doubtful. The development of a good posterior system remains a challenge. The vertebral artery is a deterrent to pedicle fixation. Do not use methylmethacrylate cement.

Halo devices

These are at best temporary and are not as reliable as a Minerva cast, but plastering skills cannot be bought like plastic halo jackets off a shelf.

Summary

I have not described operations in a catalogue fashion. That has been and will be done again elsewhere. I hope to have conveyed that surgery of the cervical spine is essentially applied anatomy. Know where you want to go. Get there slowly. Know what you want to do when you get there. It sounds simple. So is marriage. Why are there so many divorces?

Further reading

Caspar, W., Barbier, D. and Klara, P. (1989) Anterior cervical fusion and Caspar plate stabilisation for cervical trauma. *Neurosurgery*, **25**, 491–502.

Crockard, H.A. *et al.* (1986) Transoral decompression and posterior fusion for rheumatoid atlanto axial subluxation. *Journal of Bone and Joint Surgery*, **68B**, 350–356.

Mehdian, H. and Eisenstein, S. (1989) Segmental spinal instrumentation using short closed wire loops. *Clinical Orthopaedics*, **247**, 90–96.

Ransford, A.O. *et al.* (1986) Craniocervical instability treated by contoured loop fixation. *Journal of Bone and Joint Surgery*, **68B**, 173–177.

Turner, P.L. and Webb, J.K. (1987) A surgical approach to the upper thoracic spine. *Journal of Bone and Joint Surgery*, **69B**, 542–544.

Weatherley, C.R., Jaffray, D.. and O'Brien, J.P. (1986) Radical excision of an osteoblastoma of the cervical spine. *Journal of Bone and Joint Surgery*, **68B**, 325–328.

Index